OTHER FAST FACTS BOOKS

Fast Facts for the NEW NURSE PRACTITIONER: What You Really Need to Know in a Nutshell, 2e (*Aktan*)

Fast Facts for the ER NURSE: Emergency Department Orientation in a Nutshell, 3e (*Buettner*)

Fast Facts About GI AND LIVER DISEASES FOR NURSES: What APRNs Need to Know in a Nutshell (*Chaney*)

Fast Facts for the MEDICAL–SURGICAL NURSE: Clinical Orientation in a Nutshell (*Ciocco*)

Fast Facts for the NURSE PRECEPTOR: Keys to Providing a Successful Preceptorship in a Nutshell (*Ciocco*)

Fast Facts for the OPERATING ROOM NURSE: An Orientation and Care Guide in a Nutshell (*Criscitelli*)

Fast Facts for the ANTEPARTUM AND POSTPARTUM NURSE: A Nursing Orientation and Care Guide in a Nutshell (*Davidson*)

Fast Facts for the NEONATAL NURSE: A Nursing Orientation and Care Guide in a Nutshell (*Davidson*)

Fast Facts About PRESSURE ULCER CARE FOR NURSES: How to Prevent, Detect, and Resolve Them in a Nutshell (*Dziedzic*)

Fast Facts for the GERONOTOLOGY NURSE: A Nursing Care Guide in a Nutshell (*Eliopoulos*)

Fast Facts for the LONG-TERM CARE NURSE: What Nursing Home and Assisted Living Nurses Need to Know in a Nutshell (*Eliopoulos*)

Fast Facts for the CLINICAL NURSE MANAGER: Managing a Changing Workplace in a Nutshell, 2e (*Fry*)

Fast Facts for EVIDENCE-BASED PRACTICE: Implementing EBP in a Nutshell, 2e (*Godshall*)

Fast Facts About NURSING AND THE LAW: Law for Nurses in a Nutshell (*Grant, Ballard*)

Fast Facts for the L&D NURSE: Labor & Delivery Orientation in a Nutshell, 2e (*Groll*)

Fast Facts for the RADIOLOGY NURSE: An Orientation and Nursing Care Guide in a Nutshell (*Grossman*)

Fast Facts on ADOLESCENT HEALTH FOR NURSING AND HEALTH PROFESSIONALS: A Care Guide in a Nutshell (*Herrman*)

Fast Facts for the FAITH COMMUNITY NURSE: Implementing FCN/Parish Nursing in a Nutshell (*Hickman*)

Fast Facts for the CARDIAC SURGERY NURSE: Caring for Cardiac Surgery Patients in a Nutshell, 2e (*Hodge*)

Fast Facts for the CLINICAL NURSING INSTRUCTOR: Clinical Teaching in a Nutshell, 2e (*Kan, Stabler-Haas*)

Fast Facts for the WOUND CARE NURSE: Practical Wound Management in a Nutshell (*Kifer*)

Fast Facts About EKGs FOR NURSES: The Rules of Identifying EKGs in a Nutshell (*Landrum*)

Fast Facts for the CRITICAL CARE NURSE: Critical Care Nursing in a Nutshell (*Landrum*)

Fast Facts for the TRAVEL NURSE: Travel Nursing in a Nutshell (*Landrum*)

Fast Facts for the SCHOOL NURSE: School Nursing in a Nutshell, 2e (*Loschiavo*)

Fast Facts About CURRICULUM DEVELOPMENT IN NURSING: How to Develop & Evaluate Educational Programs in a Nutshell (*McCoy, Anema*)

Fast Facts for DEMENTIA CARE: What Nurses Need to Know in a Nutshell (*Miller*)

Fast Facts for HEALTH PROMOTION IN NURSING: Promoting Wellness in a Nutshell (*Miller*)

Fast Facts for STROKE CARE NURSING: An Expert Guide in a Nutshell (*Morrison*)

Fast Facts for the MEDICAL OFFICE NURSE: What You Really Need to Know in a Nutshell (*Richmeier*)

Fast Facts for the PEDIATRIC NURSE: An Orientation Guide in a Nutshell (*Rupert, Young*)

Fast Facts About the GYNECOLOGICAL EXAM FOR NURSE PRACTITIONERS: Conducting the GYN Exam in a Nutshell (*Secor, Fantasia*)

Fast Facts for the STUDENT NURSE: Nursing Student Success in a Nutshell (*Stabler-Haas*)

Fast Facts for CAREER SUCCESS IN NURSING: Making the Most of Mentoring in a Nutshell (*Vance*)

Fast Facts for the TRIAGE NURSE: An Orientation and Care Guide in a Nutshell (*Visser, (Montejano, Grossman*)

Fast Facts for DEVELOPING A NURSING ACADEMIC PORTFOLIO: What You Really Need to Know in a Nutshell (*Wittmann-Price*)

Fast Facts for the HOSPICE NURSE: A Concise Guide to End-of-Life Care (*Wright*)

Fast Facts for the CLASSROOM NURSING INSTRUCTOR: Classroom Teaching in a Nutshell (*Yoder-Wise, Kowalski*)

Fast Facts for Nurses About HOME INFUSION THERAPY: The Expert's Best Practice Guide in a Nutshell (*Gorski*)

Forthcoming FAST FACTS Books

Fast Facts About PTSD: A Clinician's Guide to Post-Traumatic Stress Disorder in a Nutshell (*Adams*)

Fast Facts on COMBATING NURSE BULLYING, INCIVILITY, AND WORKPLACE VIOLENCE: What Nurses Need to Know in a Nutshell (*Ciocco*)

Fast Facts for TESTING AND EVALUATION IN NURSING: Teaching Skills in a Nutshell (*Dusaj*)

Fast Facts About the NURSING PROFESSION: Historical Perspectives in a Nutshell (*Hunt*)

Fast Facts for the CLINICAL NURSING INSTRUCTOR: Nursing Student Success in a Nutshell, 3e (*Kan, Stabler-Haas*)

Fast Facts for the CRITICAL CARE NURSE: Critical Care Nursing in a Nutshell, 2e (*Landrum*)

Fast Facts About NURSING PATIENTS WITH MENTAL ILLNESS (MI): What RNs, NPs, and New Psych Nurses Need to Know (*Marshall*)

Fast Facts About the GYNECOLOGIC EXAM: A Professional Guide for NPs, PAs, and Midwives, 2e (*Secor, Fantasia*)

FAST FACTS for NURSES ABOUT **HOME INFUSION THERAPY**

Lisa A. Gorski, MS, RN, HHCNS-BC, CRNI®, FAAN, is a clinical nurse specialist at Wheaton Franciscan Home Health & Hospice, Milwaukee, Wisconsin. Her previous positions include surgical intensive care unit nurse and educator and adjunct faculty and clinical faculty member, University of Wisconsin. Ms. Gorski served as president of the Infusion Nurses Society (INS) 2007–2008, chaired the committee for the 2011 and 2016 INS Infusion Therapy Standards of Practice, and serves on the editorial board for *Home Healthcare Now*. She has published three books about home infusion therapy: *High Tech Home Care Manual* (1994), *Best Practices in Home Infusion Therapy* (1999), and *Pocket Guide to Home Infusion Therapy* (2005). Ms. Gorski is also coauthor of *Manual of IV Therapeutics: Evidence-Based Practice for Infusion Therapy, Sixth Edition* (2014). She is serving as the 2017–2019 Chair for the Infusion Nurses Certification Corporation and is a Fellow in the American Academy of Nursing. She speaks nationally and internationally, addressing standards development, home health care, and home infusion therapy.

FAST FACTS for NURSES ABOUT **HOME INFUSION THERAPY**

The Expert's Best-Practice Guide in a Nutshell

Lisa A. Gorski, MS, RN, HHCNS-BC, CRNI®, FAAN

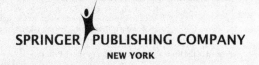

SPRINGER PUBLISHING COMPANY
NEW YORK

Copyright © 2017 Springer Publishing Company, LLC

Springer Publishing Company, LLC
11 West 42nd Street
New York, NY 10036
www.springerpub.com

Acquisitions Editor: Margaret Zuccarini
Senior Production Editor: Kris Parrish
Compositor: Westchester Publishing Services

ISBN: 978-0-8261-6005-8
e-book ISBN: 978-0-8261-6006-5

17 18 19 20 / 5 4 3 2 1

The author and the publisher of this Work have made every effort to use sources believed to be reliable to provide information that is accurate and compatible with the standards generally accepted at the time of publication. Because medical science is continually advancing, our knowledge base continues to expand. Therefore, as new information becomes available, changes in procedures become necessary. We recommend that the reader always consult current research and specific institutional policies before performing any clinical procedure. The author and publisher shall not be liable for any special, consequential, or exemplary damages resulting, in whole or in part, from the readers' use of, or reliance on, the information contained in this book. The publisher has no responsibility for the persistence or accuracy of URLs for external or third-party Internet websites referred to in this publication and does not guarantee that any content on such websites is, or will remain, accurate or appropriate.

Library of Congress Cataloging-in-Publication Data

Names: Gorski, Lisa A., author.
Title: Fast facts for nurses about home infusion therapy : the expert's best-practice guide in a
    nutshell / Lisa A. Gorski.
Other titles: Fast facts (Springer Publishing Company)
Description: New York, NY : Springer Publishing Company, LLC, [2017] | Series: Fast facts |
    Includes bibliographical references.
Identifiers: LCCN 2017000294 (print) | LCCN 2017000547 (ebook) | ISBN 9780826160058
    (hard copy : alk. paper) | ISBN 9780826160065 (ebook)
Subjects: | MESH: Home Infusion Therapy—nursing | Infusions, Parenteral—nursing
Classification: LCC RM149 (print) | LCC RM149 (ebook) | NLM WY 115.1 | DDC 615/.6—dc23
LC record available at https://lccn.loc.gov/2017000294

Printed in the United States of America by Gasch Printing.

I dedicate this book to my husband, John Connors—he has been exceedingly patient, understanding, and encouraging with all of my professional endeavors—and also to my colleagues in the Infusion Nurses Society and home care nurses everywhere who work to ensure that our patients who require infusion therapy receive the best possible care.

Contents

Reviewers

Kimberly Duff, RN, BSN

Manager, Clinical Education
Global Medical Affairs Strategy Lead in Immunology
Shire
Knoxville, Tennessee

Chris Geary, RN, BSN

Case Manager
Wheaton Franciscan Home Health & Hospice
Milwaukee, Wisconsin

Alison C. Jennings, MS, AGPCNP-BC, CRNI®

Regional Clinical Manager
Visiting Nurse Service of New York
Infusion Care Network
New York, New York

Nancy Kramer, RN, BSN, CRNI®

Vice President of Clinical Affairs
National Home Infusion Association
Alexandria, Virginia

Mary McGoldrick, MS, RN, CRNI®

Home Care and Hospice Consultant
Home Health Systems, Inc.
St. Simons Island, Georgia

Barbara Prasser, RN, BSN

Case Manager
Wheaton Franciscan Home Health & Hospice
Milwaukee, Wisconsin

Char Rondinelli, RN, BSN

Case Manager
Wheaton Franciscan Home Health & Hospice
Milwaukee, Wisconsin

Foreword

In today's health care environment, transition of care to the home is occurring at a rapid pace. Patients are receiving an array of infusion treatments ranging from a simple injection to complex intravenous infusions, and length of treatment can be days or a lifetime. Not only are all populations served, from the pediatric to the geriatric patient, but attention and education must be provided to the patient's support system: spouse, family member, or caregiver. And while infusion-related complications and untoward patient outcomes tend to occur less frequently in the home compared with the hospital, risks are still inherent in this setting. Home care nurses and the agencies that employ them must ensure they are providing safe, cost-effective patient care.

Fast Facts for Nurses About Home Infusion Therapy: The Expert's Best-Practice Guide in a Nutshell sets the stage for competent practice in Part I with a description of foundational principles of home infusion therapy, including the Gorski Model for Safe Home Infusion Therapy, nurse competency, patient education, and infection prevention concepts. The home care nurse is exposed to a variety of vascular and other access devices and it is imperative that the nurse have the critical thinking skills needed to select the appropriate vascular access device, perform or teach care and management practices, and implement strategies to prevent the development of complications. Part II covers that vital information, along with practice recommendations that are supported by the most recent available research. Part III describes proper IV delivery methods and principles for safe administration for common types of infusion therapies seen in the home.

The author clearly articulates and describes the comprehensive practice of home infusion therapy in simple terms to enable understanding and encourage ease of implementation in the nurse's practice. Features such as "Fast Facts in a Nutshell" and "Test Yourself" enhance the utility of this resource. Case studies with critical thinking questions can be used by educators and managers as part of an organizational competency program.

Infusion therapy can be delivered safely and effectively in the home setting. Successful home care agencies provide knowledgeable and qualified home care nurses and have structures and processes in place to ensure quality patient care. As an invaluable resource, this handbook can provide the framework for an effective home infusion therapy program that ensures optimal outcomes and patient safety. Every home care nurse and home care agency should include this "must have" reference in their library. Our patients deserve nothing less.

Mary Alexander, MA, RN, CRNI®, CAE, FAAN
CEO, Infusion Nurses Society
Norwood, Massachusetts

Preface

> It is a rule without any exception, that no patient ought ever to stay a day longer in hospital than is absolutely essential for medical or surgical treatment.
>
> —*Florence Nightingale, Notes on Hospitals, 1863*

Although the initial growth of home infusion began in the 1980s, escalating numbers of older adults, the increasing prevalence of chronic illnesses, and health care reform have only accelerated the need for expertly delivered home care. Although there is certainly risk for any patient living with an invasive device at home, home infusion therapy is generally a safe and common practice that allows patients to be discharged earlier from the hospital or, in some cases, avoid hospitalization altogether. Since 1985, I have worked as a clinical nurse specialist for a home care agency and have focused on the practice of home infusion therapy, providing clinical education, validating nurse competency, performing quality improvement activities, and managing many patients requiring home infusions. Home care nurses must have an up-to-date, evidence-based reference book for managing patients receiving home infusion therapy. Recognizing the continued need for a concise reference for nurses, this is my fourth book on the topic. *Fast Facts for Nurses About Home Infusion Therapy: The Expert's Best-Practice Guide in a Nutshell* is intended to meet that need.

Part I addresses the foundations of home infusion therapy. The first chapter describes my model for safe infusion therapy, which provides a framework for the subsequent chapters. This model predicts that positive outcomes, including the absence of infusion therapy–related complications, patient satisfaction, and health care provider satisfaction, are maximized when four aspects of care are addressed during the home care planning process and during the process of providing care. Chapter 2 discusses the importance of patient education. The role that patients and caregivers play in home infusion therapy is what makes home care unique. The nurse's skill in teaching patients is equally important as any infusion administration skills! The last chapter in this part describes concepts in infection prevention, an important goal of infusion therapy in all health care settings. Part II addresses access devices and methods, including peripheral catheters, the growing use of midline catheters, and central vascular access devices, as well as subcutaneous infusion and intrathecal catheters. Part III includes a chapter on infusion methods and issues followed by infusion therapy–specific chapters. Each of these chapters follows a similar format based upon my model.

Fast Facts for Nurses About Home Infusion Therapy: The Expert's Best-Practice Guide in a Nutshell is especially intended for the practicing home care nurse, to be used as a quick reference when preparing to admit patients who are receiving home infusion therapy and when out in the field seeing patients. Others who will find this book helpful include discharge planners or case managers who facilitate the transition from acute to home care, home care managers, supervisors, and educators. I hope you find this book helpful in your practice and welcome your comments and suggestions.

Lisa A. Gorski

Acknowledgments

At Springer Publishing:
Margaret Zuccarini, Publisher, who was so helpful and instrumental in bringing this book into reality

Amanda Devine, Assistant Editor, for guiding the manuscript from submission to publication

Kris Parrish, Senior Production Editor, for guiding this manuscript through the production process

Appreciation is also expressed to the following for providing illustrations and pictures:
Access Scientific
Cenorin
Halyard
Immune Deficiency Foundation
Sherry Lokken, RN, Infusion Project Manager at Omnicare

I

Foundations of Home Infusion Therapy

1

Overview and Introduction to Home Infusion Therapy

As an important aspect of U.S. health care reform, health care provided outside of the hospital setting continues to grow, and this growth is also apparent across the globe. Contributing factors include an aging population, the increasing incidence of chronic illnesses, and the continued pressure to reduce cost through reducing the incidence of hospitalizations and the length of hospital stay. The overarching goal of home care is to maintain patients safely in the home setting and prevent rehospitalization. The provision of infusion therapies in the home is a common practice that allows patients to be discharged earlier from the hospital or, potentially, to avoid hospitalizations.

Although the overall safety of home infusion therapy has been established over the past 30-some years, infusion therapy is still a "high risk" area of practice for patients who require an invasive device and may be receiving high-risk drug infusions such as antineoplastics, opioids, and inotropes. Even home intravenous (IV) antibiotic therapy can result in significant adverse events such as nephrotoxicity or ototoxicity associated with medications such as the aminoglycoside antibiotics (Gorski, 2017). Safe and effective delivery of home infusion therapy is ensured when the home care agency provides knowledgeable and qualified home care nurses and when there are structures and processes in place to ensure quality patient care.

After reading this chapter, the reader will be able to:

- Discuss four aspects of care that impact home infusion therapy outcomes
- Identify components of a successful home infusion therapy program
- Describe characteristics of a competent home infusion nurse
- Identify professional organizations relevant to home infusion therapy

Fast Facts in a Nutshell

Infusion therapy refers to the administration of solutions or medications via the IV, subcutaneous, intraosseous, and intraspinal route. The most common route is the IV route via either a peripheral or a central vascular access device (VAD). Subcutaneous and intraspinal infusions are less common routes but are also performed in the home setting. Intraosseous infusion is currently not a route for home infusion and thus not addressed in this book. Home-administered infusion therapies include antimicrobials, hydration solutions, parenteral nutrition, antineoplastic infusions, analgesics, cardiac infusion therapies for heart failure management, and immunoglobulins. A variety of other medications may be home administered as addressed in the final chapter of this book. Home infusion therapy is provided to patients across the life span.

EVIDENCE-BASED PRACTICE AND STANDARDS OF PRACTICE

The *Home Health Nursing: Scope and Standards of Practice* (American Nurses Association [ANA], 2014) provides standards for professional performance. Standard 9—Evidence-Based Practice and Research—requires the home health care nurse to "integrate evidence and research findings into practice and use current evidence-based nursing knowledge, including research findings, to guide practice" (ANA, 2014, p. 64). Although a comprehensive discussion of evidence-based practice is beyond the scope of this handbook, the concept is briefly defined and addressed. Evidence-based practice is defined as a problem-solving approach to clinical practice and administrative issues that integrates:

- A systematic search for and critical appraisal of the most relevant evidence to answer a burning clinical question
- One's own clinical expertise
- Patient preferences and values (Melnyk & Fineout-Overholt, 2014)

The Infusion Nurses Society (INS) publishes evidence-based infusion therapy practice standards approximately every 5 years. These standards are widely used and cited in the United States and across the globe (Gorski et al., 2016). The references used to support the INS recommendations are rated according to the level of evidence. The reader is referred to the standards for a discussion on the methodology and rating scale used to support the references for each recommendation. The Infusion Therapy Standards of Practice are intended to be used by clinicians in any setting where infusion therapy is administered and the standards will be frequently cited throughout this book.

THE GORSKI MODEL FOR SAFE HOME INFUSION THERAPY

The Gorski Model for Safe Home Infusion Therapy (Figure 1.1) predicts that positive outcomes, which include the absence of infusion therapy–related complications, patient satisfaction, and health care provider satisfaction, are maximized when four aspects of care are addressed during the home care planning process and during the process of providing care. This model provides a framework for Parts II and III of this book.

Fast Facts in a Nutshell

Four aspects of care that impact clinical outcomes in home infusion therapy are (a) appropriate patient selection; (b) effective patient education; (c) meticulous patient care and comprehensive assessment, and monitoring; and (d) interprofessional communication and collaboration.

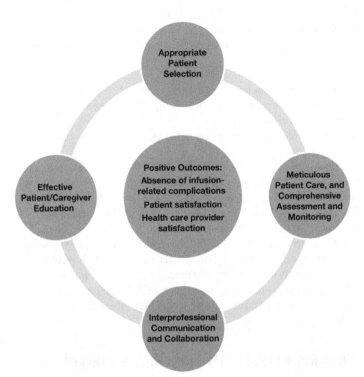

Figure 1.1 Gorski Model for Safe Home Infusion Therapy. *Source: Copyright ©*
Lisa Gorski.

The first aspect of care is *appropriate patient selection*. Patient selection criteria specific to VADs, infusion administration methods, and the type of infusion therapy are addressed in Parts II and III of this book. Some general questions to ask in terms of patient selection include:

■ Can the infusion therapy be safely administered in the home setting?
■ Is the patient and/or caregiver(s) accepting of the home care plan?
■ Is the VAD (or subcutaneous or intraspinal route) and the infusion administration method appropriate for the patient and the prescribed infusion therapy?
■ Does the home agency have competent nurses and up-to-date policies and procedures, including admission criteria, related to the type of infusion therapy that the patient requires (e.g., inotropic infusions, intraspinal infusions, and parenteral nutrition)?

- Is attention paid to the transitioning of the patient from acute to home care (e.g., patient is tolerating prescribed infusion without adverse reaction, caregiver availability as appropriate, orders for appropriate laboratory studies, and reimbursement verified and explained to the patient)?

The second aspect of care is *effective patient/caregiver education.* Patient education is especially critical to the outcome of safe infusion therapy. In most cases, the patient, or a competent caregiver, is expected to learn how to administer infusion therapy. Even in cases where most of the infusion administration–related skills are performed by the nurse (e.g., antineoplastic infusions initiated via an implanted port), the patient still must safely live with a running infusion and VAD. As addressed in the INS standards, patient education includes some level of care and maintenance of the VAD, precautions for preventing infection and other complications, use and troubleshooting of an infusion pump, and how to live with a VAD including activity limitations and activities of daily living (Gorski et al., 2016, pp. S25–S26). Patient education strategies are covered in Chapter 2 and specific topics for patient education are identified in subsequent chapters.

The third aspect of care includes *meticulous patient care and comprehensive assessment and monitoring.* Infusion administration and access device care is provided utilizing aseptic technique and sound, evidence-based procedures. This requires competent nurses, as addressed later in this chapter, with excellent assessment skills as well as expert home infusion pharmacists. The competency under the "Assessment" standard from the *Home Health Nursing: Scope and Standards of Practice* states that the nurse collects comprehensive data in a systematic and ongoing process (ANA, 2014, p. 44). A thorough baseline assessment is conducted at the first home visit. For Medicare-certified home care agencies, this will include data required on the Outcome Assessment and Information Set (OASIS). Although assessment data specific to VADs, infusion administration methods, and the type of infusion therapy are addressed in Parts II and III of this book, some general areas of assessment and monitoring during both the initial and ongoing home visits include:

- Environmental assessment including safety (e.g., electrical), structural (e.g., stairways and barriers to bedside infusion pump), and sanitation hazards (e.g., running water and refrigeration)

- Functional limitations and cognitive ability in relation to ability to learn infusion procedures, how patient best learns, caregiver/family support, and involvement in learning infusion therapy
- Vital signs, infusion access device site and patency, other signs and symptoms as appropriate to patient condition, progress toward self-care, therapeutic response, and presence of any side effects/adverse reactions
- Consideration for and attention to risks with certain patient populations; for example, physiologic differences or changes associated with pediatrics or older adults, which impact drug dosage and risk for adverse reactions

Fast Facts in a Nutshell

Although it is easy to focus on the infusion therapy aspects of assessment and become "task-oriented" in infusion administration, a holistic approach to assessment is part of the nursing process. Additional aspects of assessment are identified in the *Home Health Nursing: Scope and Standards of Practice* (ANA, 2014, p. 44), including nutritional status, psychosocial, emotional, cultural, age-related, spiritual/transpersonal, and economic assessments. Assessment and reconciliation of medications are essential. A thorough assessment provides the nurse with information to identify nursing diagnoses and develop a comprehensive plan of care.

The fourth aspect of care is *interprofessional communication and collaboration* with the patient and caregiver and with all other involved disciplines. The Scope of Service standard from the Infusion Therapy Standards of Practice states that "members of the health care team collaborate to achieve the universal goals of safe, effective, and appropriate infusion therapy" (Gorski et al., 2016, p. S13). The American Society of Health-System Pharmacists (ASHP) also emphasizes the importance of communication in home infusion therapy (ASHP, 2014). Here are some tips on communication and collaboration with specific key members of the home infusion team:

- *Home infusion pharmacist:* Communication needs include all medications taken by patient (including over-the-counter and herbal supplements), any assessment data pertinent to infusion (e.g., environmental issues, functional/cognitive limitations, and ability to safely manage home infusion therapy), laboratory results, supply needs (regular inventory of supplies and communication of needs prior to planned delivery date), therapeutic response to infusion therapy, and progress toward independence in care. The pharmacist is an important resource to the home infusion nurse for any questions or concerns related to the therapy such as side effects, adverse reactions, and administration-related questions.

- *Physician/other licensed independent practitioner (LIP):* Collaborate with MD/LIP regarding initial plan of care and plan for home visits, laboratory results, therapeutic response to infusion therapy and any adverse/side effects or evidence of VAD complications, progress toward goals, need for further home visits, and progress toward independence in care.
  - An LIP (e.g., nurse practitioner) may be allowed by state law, regulation, and organization to provide care and services without direction or supervision within the scope of the LIP license and consistent with the privileges granted by the organization.
- *Insurance case manager (as appropriate):* Communicate initial plan of care and plan for home visits, need for further home visits and rationale, and progress toward independence in care.
- *Home care agency staff:* Provide a current clinical report (including current assessment data, any areas of specific concern, progress toward goals) to supervisor and other nurses or clinical staff (e.g., physical therapist) who may be seeing patients.

COMPONENTS OF A SUCCESSFUL HOME INFUSION THERAPY PROGRAM

There must be processes and a structure in place to support delivery of safe and consistent patient care including the following:

- Written, up-to-date, and evidence-based agency policies and procedures for home infusion therapy
- Quality improvement program (e.g., surveillance, aggregation, analysis, and reporting of infections and other adverse events)

- Competent nurses and other clinicians; the competency program includes the following:
  - A comprehensive orientation program for the home infusion nurse
  - Validation of competency by "preceptors" who are also deemed competent. A variety of measurement techniques are used:
    - *Psychomotor skills:* Demonstration of skills in the home (e.g., implanted port access); simulation of skills in a "laboratory" setting (e.g., programming an infusion pump in the office)
    - *Critical thinking skills:* Clinical scenarios
    - *Knowledge:* Written tests
    - Participation in ongoing educational programs offered by the agency, seminars, and conferences (Gorski et al., 2016, p. S19)
- Tools and resources available to support home infusion nurses, patients, and families:
  - Patient educational tools (e.g., written information, videotapes)
  - Reference tools (e.g., quick reference guides for infusion pumps)
  - Electronic health records that provide cues to essential elements of documentation
  - Clinical support (e.g., clinical nurse specialist, infusion nurse specialist, home infusion pharmacist, and dietitian) available for problematic patient situations or when providing infusion therapies or infusion-related procedures new to agency staff

HOME INFUSION NURSE COMPETENCY AND KEY CHARACTERISTICS

- Highly developed clinical assessment skills, not only physical but also functional, medication-related, psychosocial, and cultural assessment (Narayan, 2011)
- Ability to effectively teach patients and caregivers
- Ability to effectively communicate and collaborate with patients, caregivers, and the interprofessional health care team
- In-depth knowledge and demonstrated competency related to infusion access devices and home infusion therapy including administration methods and potential complications
- Knowledge of community resources and reimbursement

- Good organizational and time management skills
- Ability to function independently
- Professional certification highly desirable—for example, CRNI® (certified RN—infusion therapy) by the INS

Resources for the Infusion Nurse

American Society for Parenteral and Enteral Nutrition (A.S.P.E.N.)
- An interdisciplinary professional organization focused on the science of nutritional support
- Offers certification in nutritional support
- Multiple topic standards and guidelines
- www.nutritioncare.org

Association for Professionals in Infection Control and Epidemiology (APIC)
- An interdisciplinary professional association for infection preventionists with a mission aimed at creating a safer world through the prevention of infection
- Offers certification in infection control
- www.apic.org

Association of Vascular Access (AVA)
- An interdisciplinary professional organization
- The mission of AVA is to distinguish the vascular access specialty and define standards of vascular access through an evidence-based approach designed to enhance health care
- Offers certification in vascular access
- www.avainfo.org

Immune Deficiency Foundation (IDF) Nurse Advisory Committee
- To increase awareness of primary immunodeficiency diseases through professional education and outreach on a national and international level
- Available as a resource for nurses administering immunoglobulin therapy or treating patients with primary immunodeficiency diseases
- www.primaryimmune.org/about/nurse-advisory-committee

Immunoglobulin National Society (IgNS)
- An organization dedicated to nurses and pharmacists in education, management, practice, and research in fields of immunoglobulin (Ig) therapy
- Publishes *IgNS Nursing Standards of Practice*
- Offers certification in immunoglobulin therapy
- www.ig-ns.org

Infusion Nurses Society (INS)
- A professional nursing organization focused on excellence in infusion therapy through standards, education, advocacy, and outcomes research
- Offers certification in infusion nursing
- Publishes *Infusion Therapy Standards of Practice*
- www.ins1.org

(continued)

Resources for the Infusion Nurse *(continued)*

League for Intravenous Therapy Education Vascular Access Network (LITEVAN)
- A multidisciplinary organization for networking, education, and sharing of resources related to infusion and vascular access
- www.lite.org

National Home Infusion Therapy Association (NHIA)
- A trade association that represents and advances the interests of organizations that provide infusion and specialized pharmacy services and products to the entire spectrum of home-based patients
- www.nhia.org

Oncology Nursing Society (ONS)
- A nursing organization aimed at advancing excellence in oncology nursing
- Offers certification in oncology nursing
- www.ons.org

TEST YOUR KNOWLEDGE

1. Evidence-based practice integrates research, one's clinical expertise, and:
   a. Quality improvement studies
   b. Patient values
   c. Organizational policies
   d. Patient satisfaction
2. A positive outcome in home infusion therapy, as described in the Gorski Model for Safe Home Infusion Therapy, includes:
   a. Patient satisfaction
   b. Nurse competency
   c. Effective patient education
   d. Comprehensive home care planning
3. Which of the following is required to ensure "meticulous patient care and comprehensive assessment and monitoring"?
   a. Sound patient selection criteria
   b. Highly competent nurses
   c. Effective patient educational tools
   d. An electronic health record
4. You are a former critical care nurse with 10 years of experience and have just transitioned to working in home infusion. Based on your past experience, the home care agency should:

a. Acknowledge and expect that you are competent in infusion therapy procedures
b. Ask you to be a preceptor to new nurses
c. Validate your infusion competency upon your orientation to the agency
d. Validate your competency using only a written test

ANSWERS

1. b
2. a
3. b
4. c

References

American Nurses Association. (2014). *Home health nursing: Scope and standards of practice* (2nd ed.). Silver Spring, MD: Author.

American Society of Health-System Pharmacists. (2014). ASHP guidelines on home infusion pharmacy services. *American Journal of Health-System Pharmacists, 71*, 325–341.

Gorski, L. A. (2017). The 2016 Infusion Therapy Standards. *Home Healthcare Now, 35*(1), 10–18.

Gorski, L. A., Hadaway, L., Hagle, M., McGoldrick, M., Orr, M., & Doellman, D. (2016). Infusion therapy standards of practice. *Journal of Infusion Nursing, 39*(1S), S1–S159.

Melnyk, B. M., & Fineout-Overholt, E. (2014). *Evidence-based practice in nursing and healthcare: A guide to best practice* (3rd ed.). Philadelphia, PA: Wolters Kluwer.

Narayan, M. C. (2011). Managing the complexities of home health care. In L. Neal-Boylan (Ed.), *Clinical case studies in home health care* (pp. 13–21). West Sussex, UK: John Wiley.

2

Patient Education:
An Essential Component
of Safe Home Infusion Therapy

Effective teaching is unquestionably essential to the provision of safe home infusion therapy. Patient education is one of the four aspects of care that impact patient outcomes as described in the Gorski Model for Safe Home Infusion Therapy (Chapter 1). Experienced nurses who are new to home care often enter the world of home infusion therapy confident in their own ability to administer intravenous (IV) medications and care for vascular access devices (VADs). Quickly, it becomes apparent that technical skills in infusion therapy procedures are important, but equally important is the nurse's skill in educating the patient to perform those same infusion procedures. In the majority of cases, home infusion therapy procedures are taught to and performed by patients and/or their caregivers. For example, most patients will learn to infuse their own IV antibiotics and parenteral nutrition (PN). It is important to recognize that when patients are not effectively taught, the risk for complications such as infection or adverse drug reactions is increased.

In the context of patient education, home care nurses must always assess the appropriateness of the skill being taught. Home care clinicians become very comfortable teaching patients and caregivers skills normally performed by nurses in any other health care setting. There is not a specific listing of every home infusion procedure amenable to teaching. Sometimes, issues such as insurance coverage or geographic location (e.g., rural extremes) drive decisions and push for a high level of patient participation. However, nurses must always exercise professional judgment and critical thinking skills, weigh the risks versus the benefits, and act as a patient advocate when teaching home infusion skills. For real-life situations, consider the following:

- Is it in the patient's best interest to have him or her discontinue and remove the port needle after a chemotherapy infusion? Is this a simple task or does it require assessment of response to the infusion therapy, of the port site, and for potential therapy/VAD-related complications?
- Is it appropriate for a patient or a caregiver to perform site care on a peripherally inserted central catheter (PICC) and change the stabilization device? What is the risk for PICC dislodgement? Is the patient/caregiver capable of adhering to aseptic technique with this more complex procedure?
- Is it appropriate to change administration methods (e.g., elastomeric device to gravity) without a home visit, even if the patient was independent with the previous method? What are the implications should the infusion run in too fast?

When effective teaching strategies are used with each home visit, home care is more cost-effective because fewer home visits are needed to achieve patient independence in infusion care. Most commercial insurers authorize a limited number of home visits at the start of care to teach home infusion therapy. Each visit must be used judiciously to teach patients. Some patients may require an additional visit(s) to learn infusion procedures. The home care nurse must be prepared to clearly articulate progress in patient education and describe clear rationale outlining the need for additional visits, particularly when requesting coverage or authorization of additional visits from the patient's insurer.

After reading this chapter, the reader will be able to:

- Identify factors that affect the patient's readiness to learn
- Develop a plan for patient education
- Employ effective teaching strategies
- Evaluate the effectiveness of the teaching plan

ASSESSMENT: READINESS TO LEARN

Teaching infusion therapy requires that the patient learn multistep procedures, concepts such as aseptic technique, some math skills such as counting drops or reading an infusion pump, and understanding relationships such as the importance of hand hygiene in reducing infection risk. The patient's or caregiver's readiness and ability to learn home infusion therapy are influenced by a number of factors such as current stressors, sensory deficits, and functional abilities. Past experiences with health care may positively or negatively shape attitudes toward learning. Additional factors that impact the teaching–learning process include age, developmental and cognitive level, culture and language, and health literacy (Gorski et al., 2016, p. S25). Some areas to guide assessment include:

- Presence of stresses that affect readiness/ability to learn such as:
  - Fear and anxiety over learning home infusion therapy
  - Coping with a new medical diagnosis and treatment and implications such as inability to eat normally and dependence on PN
  - Pain or weakness/fatigue from a stressful hospitalization/surgery
- Sensory deficits that impact ability; for older adults, sensory decline is a natural occurrence of the aging process.
  - A loss of elasticity in the lens of the eye results in visual changes including delayed recovery from glare, decreased ability to adapt to light, decrease in color discrimination, and difficulty in seeing small print, especially under poor lighting conditions. Furthermore, there is an increased incidence of eye diseases including glaucoma/cataracts and macular degeneration (Cacchione, 2005).
  - Age-associated changes in hearing include decreased ability to hear high-frequency sounds (e.g., alarms on an infusion pump), less ability to hear in the context of background noise, and difficulty hearing high-pitched sounds such as *s, z, sh,* and *ch* (Cacchione, 2005).
- Functional limitations such as issues with coordination, dexterity, and steadiness of hand/fingers that would affect the ability to perform infusion procedures
- Past experiences that impact learning home infusion therapy such as:
  - *Positive experience:* The patient with diabetes who has self-administered insulin may be less anxious about learning home infusion due to comfort with syringes.

- *Negative experience:* The patient who was recently hospitalized with a catheter-related bloodstream infection (CR-BSI). The caregiver who administered the PN is now afraid to perform newly prescribed home IV antibiotic infusions because he or she believes he or she caused the infection.
- Developmental and/or age-related considerations, for example:
  - Middle-aged adults may have many work and family obligations that affect timing of medication doses.
  - *Pediatric implications:* For infants, toddlers, and young children, teaching will be aimed primarily at the parent, while older children and teenagers will likely want to participate in their infusion administration.
  - Presence of memory or cognitive issues that may make teaching more challenging or could preclude the ability to learn procedures. If present, is there a willing/available caregiver and if not, is it possible/realistic for the home care nurse to administer all infusions? Normal changes in cognition associated with aging include reduced processing speed, tendency to be distracted, and reduced capacity to process and remember new information at the same time (U.S. Department of Health and Human Services, n.d.-a).
  - Culturally pertinent implications related to learning such as religious preferences, involvement of family/caregiver in care, attitudes toward medications and health care practices, and need for language interpretation services.
- Health literacy:
  - Health literacy refers to the degree to which individuals have the capacity to obtain, process, and understand basic health information and services needed to make appropriate health decisions (U.S. Department of Health and Human Services, n.d.-b).

Fast Facts in a Nutshell

Health literacy includes basic ability to read, knowledge of health topics, and number skills. The American Nurses Association's (ANA) Professional Performance Standard on Communication addresses the importance of assessing language and literacy needs of patients in learning how to best communicate (ANA, 2014, p. 67).

PLANNING PATIENT EDUCATION

- Plan interventions based upon issues identified from baseline assessment. Some examples might include addressing pain issues, timing home visits and infusions with attention to patient's need for sleep and rest, and providing an environment conducive to teaching (reduce background noise, good lighting).
- Plan teaching strategies based on how patient best learns. Recognize that, even for patients who are highly literate, some may prefer to learn by observing and doing than by reading; many persons who are not able to read well will hide this fact, and would benefit from pictured, step-by-step instructions.
- Establish teaching goals *with* the patient/caregiver and within the anticipated duration of home care:
  - Address reimbursement issues that affect the plan (does the patient's insurer pay for a limited number of home visits? Is there a significant copayment for each visit?).
- Plan frequency of home visits—usually based upon frequency of home infusion therapy administration.
- Encourage patient and/or caregiver to discuss concerns and anxieties related to plan for home infusion therapy.
- Enlist the help of a caregiver, if appropriate, to assist with or perform infusion procedures.
- Use educational resources that are understandable. Incorporate any agency tools (e.g., pathways, standardized teaching plans, or checklists) and patient education handouts as appropriate. Teaching topics specific to VADs and infusion therapies are discussed in subsequent chapters.
- Ensure that any websites used are reputable and advise patients about the benefits and challenges associated with social media when used to obtain health advice and information and social support (Gorski et al., 2016, p. S25). Safety, privacy, and misinformation are challenges associated with both websites and social media sites.

Fast Facts in a Nutshell

Schedule home infusion therapy and teaching sessions to meet the patient's needs. For example, some patients may do much better with a daily noon dose of IV antibiotic instead of an 8 a.m. dose. A gradual change in administration time may be needed to ensure consistent serum drug levels; collaborate with pharmacist and physician in making any changes to the medication schedule.

IMPLEMENTATION: PATIENT EDUCATION STRATEGIES

- Be sensitive to the anxiety and fears that many patients and caregivers may have in relation to administering medications into a catheter that is "near the heart."
- Ensure that the environment is conducive to teaching with good lighting and minimal noise.
- Foster an unhurried and relaxed atmosphere.
- Use a slower pace of teaching if needed, especially when working with older adults.
- Make direct eye contact. Be alert to facial expressions that indicate a lack of understanding. Use "plain language" avoiding medical jargon and vague terms.
- Use "teach-back" technique (see Table 2.1).
- Provide good-quality written instructions:
  - Written materials should be at the fifth- to seventh-grade reading level; there are various readability formulas available; most word processing programs can calculate grade level and readability.
  - Other factors that improve readability include large font size (at least 12–13 point font); avoiding use of all capital letters; format; use of illustrations; and color of type and paper (e.g., black type on yellow paper is easy to read; Doak, Doak, & Root, 1996).
  - Keep sentences short, use plain language, and be specific and direct (Foster, Idossa, Mau, & Murphy, 2016).
  - Written instructions should be available in additional languages, based on the populations served by the home care agency.
  - Some patients may prefer to write procedural steps in their own words.

Table 2.1

Using Teach-Back Technique

- Use plain and simple language avoiding jargon, complex medical terms, and most acronyms. An exception might be the frequently used acronym PICC, for "peripherally inserted central catheter," which is understood by most patients after teaching.
- Provide explanations of procedures and clearly demonstrate steps.
- Teach procedures in small portions; for example, focus on flushing procedures first; when mastered, move on to setting up the infusion tubing/priming.
- Focus on "need-to-know" information and emphasize key points.
- Simplify steps whenever possible.
- Ask patients to repeat instructions in their own words, to demonstrate skills back to the nurse.
- Clarify and correct information if patient is unable to "teach-back" correctly. Repeat and rephrase information as necessary to increase understanding. This may take several times.

Source: Kornberger, Gibson, Sadowski, Maletta, and Kingeil (2013).

- Be creative! Help patients make associations between infusion therapy and other day-to-day activities such as:
  - Changing the battery in an infusion pump is like changing the battery in another portable gadget that the patient uses.
  - Resetting the infusion pump is similar to punching in the settings on a microwave oven.

Fast Facts in a Nutshell

Plain language makes it easier for everyone to understand and use health information. Some examples are as follows:

Instead of "associated with," say "goes along with" or "happens with"
Instead of "bacteria," say "germs"
Instead of "contaminated," say "not clean" or "dirty"
Instead of "disease," say "sickness" (Centers for Disease Control and Prevention [CDC], 2016)

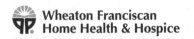

Wheaton Franciscan
Home Health & Hospice

Home Infusion Therapy Program: Patient Teaching Certificate

Patient name: _____
Caregiver name: _____
Type of infusion therapy: _____
Name of infusion pump: _____
Infusion pharmacy: _____

1. I have been taught and have shown my nurse that I know how to:
   (check those that apply) Care for my intravenous (IV) catheter:
   ( ) Change the dressing
   ( ) Change the cap
   ( ) Flush with heparin and/or saline
2. Give my own IV medicine:
   ( ) Store medicine and supplies properly
   ( ) Set up equipment
   ( ) Manage the IV pump
   ( ) Maintain sterile technique
   ( ) Dispose of medicine and syringes and other supplies properly
   ( ) Order supplies from the infusion pharmacy
3. Identify potential complications:
   ( ) Of the IV catheter
   ( ) Of the medicine(s)
   ( ) Of the IV pump
4. Call for help or questions:
   ( ) Doctor: Name: _____ Number: _____
   ( ) Home care nurse: Name: _____ Number: _____
   ( ) Infusion pharmacy: Name: _____ Number: _____

I understand that I will administer my own IV therapy and will call my nurse, doctor, or pharmacy if I have any problems or questions.

Patient signature: _____ Date: _____
Caregiver signature: _____ Relationship: _____
Nurse signature: _____ Date: _____

Figure 2.1 Example of a patient "teaching certificate." *Source: Courtesy of Wheaton Franciscan Home Health & Hospice, Milwaukee, WI.*

A kitchen table is often an excellent location for infusion therapy teaching. There is usually good overhead lighting and comfortable seating. The table can be cleaned, a barrier laid down, and supplies can be organized in the patient's visual field and placed in the order of use.

EVALUATION OF LEARNING

- Assess progress toward learning with each home visit.
- See Table 2.1: Using Teach-Back Technique.
- Because of safety and infection control concerns with IV therapy, aseptic technique and precise skills are necessary; address any breaches in technique.
- For patients who achieve independence in administration of their infusions, it may be helpful to have the patient or caregiver sign a patient education "certificate" (Figure 2.1); this type of form is helpful in clearly outlining patient/caregiver responsibilities for care and patient acknowledgement of instructions received.
- For patients who are having difficulty learning infusion procedures, reevaluate overall plan and potential areas for improvement or a need to change the plan (see Table 2.2 for suggestions).

Table 2.2

Evaluation Questions: Patients Who Exhibit Difficulty or Inability to Learn Infusion Procedures

- Are effective teaching strategies implemented including use of "teach-back" and simple, plain language?
- Is there consistency in how the home care nurse(s) have instructed the patient? If several nurses are involved in providing home care, is everyone implementing the teaching plan and providing the patient with consistent information and feedback?
- What are the issues that are affecting ability to learn? Anxiety? Functional limitations (e.g., hand tremors impact ability to maintain aseptic technique)? Cognitive limitations? Lack of motivation? Unresolved pain? Distractions in the home? Are additional home visits likely to result in a positive outcome? Can you advocate for additional home visits with the insurance company?

(continued)

Table 2.2

Evaluation Questions: Patients Who Exhibit Difficulty or Inability to Learn Infusion Procedures *(continued)*

- Could procedures be simplified (e.g., prefilled syringes and elastomeric infusion pump)?
- Could a caregiver become more involved?
- If cognitive limitations (e.g., forgetfulness and inability to problem solve) are issues, is it possible for the home care nurse to provide all of the infusions?
- Is another infusion setting more appropriate (e.g., outpatient)?

TEST YOUR KNOWLEDGE

1. Health literacy includes:
   a. Learning multistep procedures
   b. Number skills
   c. Reading at a high school level
   d. Teaching strategies
2. Sensory changes associated with aging include:
   a. A decrease in ability to hear low-frequency sounds
   b. A more elastic eye lens
   c. Difficulty hearing high-pitched sounds such as *f* and *g*
   d. A decrease in ability to discriminate colors
3. Plain language incorporates:
   a. Use of common health care acronyms
   b. Use of common health care jargon
   c. Avoidance of vague terms
   d. Use of elementary school terms
4. An effective teaching strategy is to:
   a. Provide written handouts using capital letters
   b. Provide handouts written at the fourth-grade or lower level
   c. Include illustrations in written handouts
   d. Avoid written handouts when teaching older adults
5. Mrs. Deer is struggling to learn how to administer her IV antibiotics. You should:
   a. Suggest that another nurse provide Mrs. Deer's teaching
   b. Call the physician to obtain an order for outpatient IV administration

c. Evaluate the issues that are causing Mrs. Deer's struggles
d. Talk to the infusion pharmacist for advice
6. Critical thinking: The husband was independent with administering his wife's PN. She develops a CR-BSI, is hospitalized, and
is now back home on three times per day IV antibiotics. The
husband now refuses to administer the IV antibiotics for fear of
causing another infection. The home care nurse should:
a. Acknowledge the husband's fears and tell him that it is best
that the nurse now administer the IVs
b. Instruct that he did not cause the infection and should
administer the IVs
c. Provide education related to potential contributing factors to
the CR-BSI and plan to reevaluate the husband's technique
and provide reteaching as needed
d. Ask the insurance case manager what to do

ANSWERS

1. b
2. d
3. c
4. c
5. c
6. c

References

American Nurses Association. (2014). *Home health nursing: Scope and standards of practice* (2nd ed.). Silver Spring, MD: Author.

Cacchione, P. Z. (2005). Sensory changes. Retrieved from https://consultgeri
.org/geriatric-topics/sensory-changes

Centers for Disease Control and Prevention. (2016). Everyday words for pub-
lic health communication. Retrieved from http://www.cdc.gov/other/
pdf/everydaywords-060216-final.pdf

Doak, C. C., Doak, L. G., & Root, J. H. (1996). *Teaching patients with low literacy skills*. Philadelphia, PA: Lippincott.

Foster, J., Idossa, L., Mau, L., & Murphy, E. (2016). Applying health literacy
principles: Strategies and tools to develop easy-to-read patient education
resources. *Clinical Journal of Oncology Nursing, 20*(4), 433–436.

Gorski, L. A., Hadaway, L., Hagle, M., McGoldrick, M., Orr, M., & Doellman, D. (2016). Infusion therapy standards of practice. *Journal of Infusion
Nursing, 39*(1S), S1–S159.

Kornberger, C., Gibson, C., Sadowski, S., Maletta, K., & Kingeil, C. (2013). Using "teach-back" to promote a safe transition from hospital to home: An evidence-based approach to improving the discharge process. *Journal of Pediatric Nursing, 28*, 282–291.

U.S. Department of Health and Human Services. (n.d.-a). Quick guide to health literacy and older adults. Retrieved from https://health.gov/commu nication/literacy/olderadults/literacy.htm

U.S. Department of Health and Human Services. (n.d.-b). Quick guide to health literacy [Fact sheet]. Retrieved from https://health.gov/communi cation/literacy/quickguide/factsbasic.htm

3

Infection Prevention Concepts

Bloodstream infections (BSIs) associated with vascular access devices (VADs) are preventable. For acute care hospitals, central line–associated BSI (CLABSI) rates are publicly reported on the Medicare.gov website ("hospital compare") and *any* VAD-related BSI is considered a preventable event with treatment not reimbursable under Medicare. Although the same reporting and reimbursement constraints do not currently apply in home care, prevention of infusion-related complications, including infection, is a growing concern. For home care agencies certified by the Centers for Medicare and Medicaid (CMS), acute care hospitalizations for home care patients are publicly reported ("home care compare"). Data from the Medicare-required Outcome and Assessment Information Set (OASIS) were used to describe rates of hospitalization and emergency care use caused by infection based on a 20% random sampling of 2010 OASIS data (Shang, Larson, Liu, & Stone, 2015). Of 36,330 unplanned hospitalizations based on a sample of 199,462 patients representing 8,200 home care agencies, 17% (*n* = 1,587) of hospitalizations were due to infections with 0.3% (*n* = 105) caused by intravenous (IV) catheter-related infection. Significant characteristics associated with infections included younger age, more likely men, more likely White, had cancer or renal disease, and *more likely to be receiving IV therapy or parenteral nutrition (PN)*. A limitation of OASIS data is that the home care clinician completes the reason for hospitalization based on the best information available at the time of hospital transfer. Nevertheless, infections occur in the home care setting, are a serious problem, and considerable variation in infection control policies and practices exists (Shang et al., 2015).

After reading this chapter, the reader will be able to:

- Discuss the importance of identifying and reporting infections in home care
- Describe the pathogenesis of a catheter-related BSI
- Apply standard and transmission-based precautions in home care
- Identify specific strategies aimed at preventing infections during infusion therapy

DEFINING INFECTIONS AND CLARIFYING COMMON TERMINOLOGY

The terms *catheter-related bloodstream infection* (CR-BSI) and *central line–associated bloodstream infection* (CLABSI) are often used interchangeably, but they have different meanings. CR-BSI is a clinical diagnostic definition that requires specific laboratory testing that identifies the catheter as the source of the BSI; removal of the VAD and culturing of the catheter tip are recommended as part of the diagnostic process, from which a treatment plan can be developed. CLABSI is a surveillance definition that seeks to compare rates of infection within a population, and is defined as a primary BSI (i.e., no apparent infection at another site) that develops in a patient with a central line in place within the 48-hour period before onset of the BSI that is not related to another site; blood cultures are required (Association of Professionals in Infection Control and Epidemiology [APIC], 2015; O'Grady et al., 2011). Note that there are home care infection definitions as established by APIC and the Centers for Disease Control and Prevention's (CDC) Healthcare Infection Control Practices Advisory Committee (HICPAC; 2008), but they have not been widely applied. Home care and home hospice health care–associated infections (HAIs) include infections that were neither present nor incubating at the time of initiation of care in the patient's place of residence. Should the infection appear in a patient within 48 hours of discharge from a health care facility, the infection(s) is reported back to the facility that discharged the patient prior to his or her home care services, and thus not reported as a home care–associated infection (APIC and HICPAC, 2008).

INFECTION SURVEILLANCE IN HOME CARE

In general, the risk of infection for patients living at home with VADs or other access devices is accepted to be low. A major advantage to home infusion therapy is that the risk of transmission associated with multiple patients and multiple providers in an institution is eliminated in the home setting. Some patients, however, may face increased risk for infection due to such factors as being immunocompromised (e.g., pediatric oncology patients), having a multilumen VAD, or receiving a higher risk infusion such as PN (Buchman, Opilla, Kwasny, Diamantidis, & Okamoto, 2014; Gorski et al., 2016; Keller et al., 2016; Rinke, Milstone, et al., 2013; Shang, Ma, Poghosyan, Dowding, & Stone, 2014). Patient and caregiver self-administration of infusions may pose a potential risk; however, this may also be an advantage for the many patients who take their role in performing their infusions and VAD care very seriously. Environmental factors have been hypothesized as risk factors for infections. Common exposures including well water, cooking with raw meat, soil exposure through yard work, or having a pet in the home were not found to increase the risk of central VAD (CVAD) complications in a recent prospective study (Keller et al., 2016).

In an 11-year surveillance study from the University of North Carolina Health Care System, the overall rate of home care CLABSI was very low at 0.22 infections per 1,000 device days representing nine infections over 40,763 device days (Weber, Brown, Huslage, Sickber-Bennett, & Rutala, 2009). The cases were identified by home care nurses and reviewed by infection control staff using CDC definitions of nosocomial infections. Ask yourself the following questions in relation to *your* home care organization:

- Do you know what the CLABSI rate is in your home care organization?
- Do you report possible catheter-related infections as part of your agency's performance improvement program?

Unlike acute care hospitals, in home care the reality is that infection surveillance is not consistently performed and infection rates are not consistently measured or not measured consistently with standardized surveillance definitions. Challenges include ensuring a reliable reporting system, calculating VAD days, and validating infections. In an investigation of home care agency CLABSI definitions and prevention policies in pediatric home care, only 25% (14/57) of surveyed agencies knew their overall CLABSI rate (mean 0.40 CLABSIs per 1,000 central line days; Rinke, Bundy, et al., 2013).

Despite the challenges, without identifying and tracking infections, it is difficult to identify areas for performance improvement. Home care agencies must strive to do better. Helpful strategies and tools for data collection are published in a "toolkit" available online (United Hospital Fund, 2016). When an agency does identify infection rates, opportunities for improvement are identified. Consider the following example:

Infections in patients with PICCs [peripherally inserted central catheters] were reduced by 46% in patients receiving home infusions (0.963 to 0.52 infections per 1000 central line days). A lack of standardized care protocols was identified as a key problem and interventions included standardizing home health central line orders (NC [needleless connector] changing and disinfection, flushing, blood draws, site care), development of checklists for central line care and flushing, and nursing education. (Baumgarten et al., 2013)

Fast Facts in a Nutshell

VAD-related infections that occur in a home care patient must be considered *potentially preventable*. Any infection that occurs should result in a case review by the clinicians involved in the case. Areas to discuss include patient risk factors (e.g., high-risk infusions such as PN, immunocompromised status, and type of VAD including number of lumens), environmental factors (e.g., cleanliness of home and pets), nursing adherence to infection prevention practices, and patient teaching strategies and evaluation of their effectiveness. Although it is easy to place "blame" on a patient and/or the home situation, a critical and objective look at agency practices, in hindsight, may uncover opportunities for improvement and risk reduction.

PATHOGENESIS OF CR-BSIs

Microorganisms gain access to the vascular system, potentially leading to a BSI via four main routes: extraluminal, intraluminal,

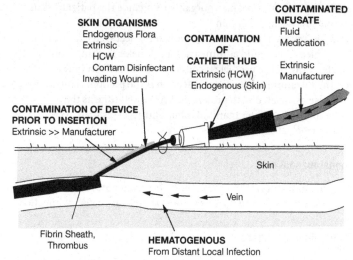

SKIN ORGANISMS
Endogenous Flora
Extrinsic
    HCW
    Contam Disinfectant
    Invading Wound

**CONTAMINATION
OF
CATHETER HUB**
Extrinsic (HCW)
Endogenous (Skin)

**CONTAMINATED
INFUSATE**
Fluid
Medication

Extrinsic
Manufacturer

**CONTAMINATION OF DEVICE
PRIOR TO INSERTION**
Extrinsic >> Manufacturer

Skin

Vein

Fibrin Sheath,
Thrombus

HEMATOGENOUS
From Distant Local Infection

Figure 3.1 Sources of IV-related infections. *Source: Safdar et al. (2014). Used with permission.*

HCW, health care worker.

hematogenous seeding, and through contaminated infusate (APIC, 2015; O'Grady et al., 2011; Safdar, Maki, & Mermel, 2014; see Figure 3.1).

Extraluminal

Organisms at the insertion site or on a contaminated catheter migrate into the catheter tract and along the external catheter surface, thus gaining access to vascular system.

■ Potential sources of microorganisms include the patient's skin, health care worker (HCW)/caregiver hands, or contaminated disinfectant.
■ The extraluminal source for infection is the predominant cause in the short term (e.g., within the first 2 weeks after VAD insertion; Mermel, 2011).

Intraluminal

Direct contamination of the catheter or catheter hub occurs, giving microorganisms access through the internal lumen of the catheter.

- Potential sources of microorganisms include the patient's skin and HCW/caregiver hands.
- Risk is present every time the catheter is accessed (e.g., during medication or fluid administration, catheter flushing, and changing of the needleless connector [NC] or IV tubing).
- The intraluminal source of infection is the predominant cause associated with prolonged VAD dwell time as the number of catheter manipulations and accesses increases (Mermel, 2011).

Hematogenous

Organisms are carried to the catheter from a remote source of infection present in the patient. This is considered a rare cause of infection.

Contaminated Infusate

- *Intrinsic contamination:* Infusates can become contaminated during the manufacturing process. This is a rare cause of infection; however, it can cause epidemic device-related infections because of the large numbers of patients in multiple settings who may be affected.
- *Extrinsic contamination:* Risk is present if infusates are not properly handled (e.g., improper refrigeration, failure to adhere to aseptic technique during solution preparation).

STRATEGIES TO REDUCE THE RISK FOR INFECTION

Always Apply Standard and Transmission-Based Precautions

Standard precautions are required in the care of all patients regardless of their infection status to protect the clinician as well as the patient. Standard precautions are based on the principle that all blood, body fluids, secretions and excretions (except sweat), nonintact skin, and mucous membranes may contain transmissible infectious agents. Standard precautions are intended to protect the health care provider as well as the patient from health care–associated transmission of infectious agents (Siegel, Rhinehart, Jackson, & Chiarello, 2007). Standard precautions include the following infection prevention practices: hand hygiene; personal protective equipment (PPE), such as gloves, gowns, masks, eye protection, or face shields; and safe injection practices.

Fast Facts in a Nutshell

Nurses should have PPE readily available during the course of making home visits. Minimally, this should include one full gown, one set of eye protection, nonsterile gloves, one face mask, and if applicable, one N95 respirator, and one resuscitation mask (McGoldrick, 2016).

Transmission-based precautions are additional precautions based on the known or suspected infectious state of the patient and the possible routes of transmission. There are exceptions to application of transmission-based precautions, particularly in the home setting, where the risk of transmission is not well defined, an isolation room is not possible, and family members already exposed to diseases generally do not wear masks. Transmission-based precautions must be adapted and applied as appropriate in home care. There are three categories of transmission-based precautions (Siegel et al., 2007):

- *Airborne precautions* require special air handling and ventilation to prevent the spread of organisms. In the home setting, control of air handling is not possible. Clinicians caring for the patient on airborne precautions wear a mask or respirator (HEPA or N95 respirators), which is donned when entering the home setting. Although airborne precautions are not a common home infusion therapy situation, an example would be the patient with tuberculosis who is multidrug resistant and requires antimicrobial infusion therapy.
- *Droplet precautions* require the use of mucous membrane protection (eye protection and masks) to prevent infectious organisms from contacting the conjunctivae or mucous membranes of the nose or mouth. Examples of infections are mumps, rubella, influenza, adenovirus, rhinovirus, and pertussis.
- *Contact precautions* require the use of gloves and gowns when direct skin-to-skin contact or contact with a contaminated environment is anticipated. Application of contact precautions is not uncommon in home care because there are many patients with infections such as *Clostridium difficile* and infections due to multidrug resistant organisms (MDROs) such as methicillin-resistant *staphylococcus aureus* (MRSA) and vancomycin-resistant *Enterococcus* (VRE).

Fast Facts in a Nutshell

When caring for a patient with an MDRO, limit reusable patient care equipment (e.g., use disposable equipment whenever possible such as a blood pressure cuff and stethoscope) and leave in the home until discharged. Clean and disinfect before removing from the home or transport in a container to an appropriate site for cleaning and disinfection (Gorski et al., 2016; Siegel et al., 2007).

Employ Aseptic Technique: What Does This Mean?

Aseptic technique is followed for all clinical procedures associated with risk for infections, which certainly includes all infusion procedures. Confusion and misunderstanding about terminology abound!

Take the example of peripheral IV site preparation. *Clean* skin is achieved with soap and water cleansing. This would be inadequate alone for IV catheter placement. Skin antisepsis is also performed to minimize the presence of microbes on the skin prior to insertion, thus reducing risk for infection. (Phillips & Gorski, 2014)

Once a package is opened and sterile supplies are exposed to the air, the term *aseptic technique* is used, in preference to sterile technique. Aseptic technique is defined as a primary infection prevention method to maintain objects and areas maximally free from microorganisms through use of sterile supplies, barrier, and absolute separation of sterile items from those that are not sterile (Gorski et al., 2016, p. S146). Aseptic no-touch technique (ANTT) is a specific type of aseptic technique widely used throughout the United Kingdom (Rowley, Clare, Macqueen, & Molyneux, 2010). Based on a theoretical and practice framework, hand hygiene and presence of an aseptic field promote aseptic technique, but effective "no-touch" technique ensures it. Teaching patients and families to apply the principles of ANTT demonstrated success in terms of low CR-BSI incidence in a study of children who required PN (Mutalib, Evans, Hughes, & Hill, 2015). A basic principle of ANTT is that key parts of the supplies used for an infusion must not be touched, whether with or without gloves, to ensure asepsis. Following are some examples:

- The peripheral catheter, once taken out of the package and its protective covering removed, cannot be touched before insertion.
- The tip of the flush syringe is protected by a cap that is not to be removed until it is ready for use. The syringe tip is never touched prior to insertion into the NC.
- The male luer end of the administration set must be protected by a cap and not touched prior to insertion into the NC or the VAD.
- NCs must be appropriately disinfected prior to access.

The "Nurse's Bag": A Potential Source for Microbial Transmission

The home care nurse's bag can be hand-carried bags, those with shoulder straps, rolling bags, fanny packs, and/or backpacks. Always consider the potential risk for transmission of infection from one patient to another via a contaminated nurse's bag as it is carried from home to home with supplies such as blood pressure cuffs, stethoscopes, and extra supplies. Researchers cultured nurses' bags from four different home care agencies with the following results:

- *Outside of bags:* 83.6% were contaminated with human pathogens with 15.9% culturing MDROs.
- *Inside of bags:* 48.4% contamination (6.3% MDROs).
- *Patient care equipment:* 43.7% contamination (5.6% MDROs) (Bakunas-Kennely & Madigan, 2009)

Suggestions for reducing the risk of transmission associated with nurse's bags include the following:

- Perform hand hygiene before entering the bag.
- Place bag in the home on a visibly clean surface or hang on a doorknob or back of a heavy chair; placement of the bag upon a barrier (e.g., plastic bag and poly-backed towels) is controversial but consider the fact that human pathogens do survive on environmental surfaces and patient homes are not typically disinfected.
- Clean and disinfect bag regularly; suggestion of weekly; select bags that are easily cleaned (e.g., nonporous and nonfabric).

- Consider an organizational policy to clean equipment before returning it to the bag after each use.
- Place the nursing bag in the car on a visibly clean surface.
- Do not bring the bag into the homes of patients with MDROs, patients on contact precautions, in the presence of infestations, and in grossly contaminated homes. (McGoldrick, 2014)

Key Points: Reduce Risk During VAD Insertion

- Perform proper hand hygiene.
- Adhere to aseptic technique during all aspects of catheter placement.
- Promptly dispose of and replace a product should there be any break in aseptic technique.
- Clean skin if visibly dirty prior to skin antisepsis.
- Remove excess hair as needed to facilitate dressing adherence; use a scissors, never shave.
- Perform skin antisepsis; chlorhexidine in alcohol solution > 0.5% is the preferred skin antiseptic agent; if contraindicated, povidone-iodine, 70% alcohol, or tincture of iodine may be used.
- Allow antiseptic solution to fully dry, naturally.
- Use a dedicated tourniquet.
- *Short peripheral catheter (SPC) placement:* Use disposable nonsterile gloves in conjunction with a no-touch technique; the insertion site is not palpated after skin antisepsis; Infusion Nurses Society (INS) suggests increased attention to technique during placement including use of sterile gloves (Gorski et al., 2016, p. S65).
- *Central line placement* (less common in home care; in some areas, PICCs are placed in the home by trained and competent nurses): Implement the central line bundle that includes hand hygiene, chlorhexidine skin antisepsis, maximal sterile barrier protection (mask, sterile gloves/gown, cap, eye protection, and large/full body drape), and avoidance of the femoral vein in obese adults. Recommendations also include observation and completion of a checklist by an educated health care clinician, empowering the clinician to stop the procedure if any breaches in technique occur (Gorski et al., 2016, p. S65).

Reducing Risk During VAD Dwell Time: Postinsertion Care and Maintenance

- Perform proper hand hygiene prior to each aspect of VAD access or care.
- Inspect entire infusion system from solution container to the VAD for integrity of the system, infusion accuracy, and expiration dates (infusate, dressing, and administration set).
- Routine site care:
  - Skin antisepsis as a component of routine VAD site care; chlorhexidine in alcohol solution >0.5% is the preferred skin antiseptic agent.
- Dressing changes:
  - Change transparent semipermeable membrane (TSM) dressings at least every 7 days and, if using a gauze dressing, change every 2 days. Also, perform site care and change dressing earlier (i.e., as needed) if not intact, if drainage or moisture is present under the dressing. Failure to do so allows for growth of skin organisms, thus increasing the risk for infection.
  - Chlorhexidine dressings are widely used in acute care as an effective and evidence-based strategy to reduce risk for BSI with CVADs. They are most beneficial when the extraluminal route is the primary source of infection (first 2 weeks following VAD placement). The benefit and usage of such dressings in long-term and home care has not been studied; some home care organizations, however, do routinely use them, particularly with PICC lines (which do not form a "healed" or closed tract or tunnel within 2 weeks of insertion, as happens with tunneled CVADs).
- Maintain catheter patency:
  - If the flow is sluggish, or there is an inability to flush or obtain blood return in a CVAD, problem solve potential causes. If assessed as a likely thrombotic problem, obtain order to use a thrombolytic agent.
  - The presence of blood in and around the catheter/tip is a source for bacterial growth.
- NC disinfection:
  - Disinfect prior to each entry into the device using a vigorous mechanical scrub and allow to dry.
  - Acceptable disinfectants include 70% alcohol, povidone-iodine, and chlorhexidine in alcohol solution.

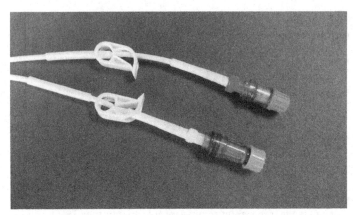

Figure 3.2 Examples of passive disinfection caps: Caps are attached to the tip of the needleless connector.

  ▪ Disinfection may not be necessary if the NC is covered with a "passive disinfection cap" (Figure 3.2) that contains a disinfectant agent (typically alcohol); these caps are discarded after removal and a fresh cap placed after completion of the intermittent infusion. The INS suggests that with each subsequent entry through the NC, a disinfectant scrub for 5 to 15 seconds should be done (Gorski et al., 2016, p. S69).
▪ VAD removal when no longer necessary:
  ▪ Any VAD is a potential source for microbial entry and should be removed if no longer needed (Gorski et al., 2016).

KEY POINTS: PATIENT EDUCATION

▪ Hand hygiene, aseptic technique, disinfection of NCs
▪ Preparation of clean work area (e.g., kitchen table) and place/organize all needed supplies for each infusion
▪ Site protection; keeping VAD dressing/tubing dry during bathing; using a designated product or plastic wrap (Figure 3.3)
▪ Storage of infusion supplies in a clean, dry, and safe area
▪ What/how to and whom to report: Signs of possible infection including redness at the site, swelling, hardness at the site, fever, and chills

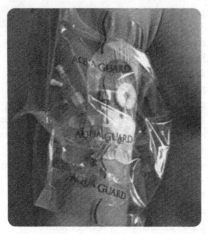

Figure 3.3 Aquaguard product (used to keep VAD dry during bathing).
Source: Courtesy of Cenorin, LLC, Kent, WA.

VAD, vascular access device.

TEST YOUR KNOWLEDGE

1. Patients who may be at higher risk for infection during home infusion therapy include:
   a. Adult patients who receive home chemotherapy
   b. Any patients who receive IV antibiotics
   c. Patients who receive home PN
   d. Patients who receive infusions via implanted ports
2. A common route for microorganisms to gain entry to the vascular system is:
   a. Via the infusate
   b. Via hematogenous seeding
   c. Via the intraluminal route
   d. Via intrinsic contamination
3. Any VAD-related infection that occurs in a home care patient:
   a. Is usually not preventable due to the patient involvement
   b. Must be considered potentially preventable
   c. Is always considered preventable
   d. Results in lost reimbursement to the home care organization
4. Early VAD-related BSI is more likely due to the entry of microorganisms via which route?
   a. Intraluminal
   b. Extraluminal

c. Hematogenous
d. Contaminated infusate
5. Aseptic technique includes:
   a. Use of clean gloves for all infusion procedures
   b. Always shaving skin before catheter placement
   c. Disinfection of the needleless connector prior to each access
   d. Cleaning skin with soap and water prior to SPC placement
6. The risk of microbial transmission from home to home may be reduced through effective handling of the nurse's bag. Recommendations include:
   a. Performing hand hygiene prior to each entry into the bag to retrieve supplies
   b. Storing the bag inside a plastic container
   c. Using nurse's bags made of a cloth material
   d. Cleaning and disinfecting the bag monthly
7. In relation to the use of chlorhexidine dressings in home care:
   a. They are routinely recommended for home care patients
   b. They reduce the risk of microbial entry via the intraluminal route
   c. Their routine use is not studied in long-term VAD use/home care
   d. They are associated with a high risk of skin reactions
8. Effective infection prevention strategies associated with NC use include:
   a. Disinfection only before the initial saline flush
   b. Allowing the disinfectant to dry before attaching the flush syringe
   c. Preferential use of chlorhexidine in alcohol for disinfection
   d. Avoiding use of passive infection caps

ANSWERS

1. c
2. c
3. b
4. b
5. c
6. a
7. c
8. b

References

Association of Professionals in Infection Control and Epidemiology. (2015). APIC implementation guide: Guide to preventing central line-associated bloodstream infections. Retrieved from http://apic.org/Resource_/Tiny MceFileManager/2015/APIC_CLABSI_WEB.pdf

Association of Professionals in Infection Control and Epidemiology and Healthcare Infection Control Practices Advisory Committee. (2008). APIC-HICPAC surveillance definitions for home health care and home hospice infections. Retrieved from http://nosobase.chu-lyon.fr/recom mandations/cdc/2008_HAD_APIC_HICPAC.pdf

Bakunas-Kennely, I., & Madigan, E. A. (2009). Infection prevention and control in home health care: The nurse's bag. *American Journal of Infection Control*, 37(8), 687–688.

Baumgarten, K., Hale, Y., Messonnier, M., McCabe, M., Albright, M., & Bergeron, E. (2013). Bridging the gap: A collaborative to reduce peripherally inserted central catheter infections in the home care environment. *The Ochsner Journal*, 13, 352–358.

Buchman, A. L., Opilla, M., Kwasny, M., Diamantidis, T. G., & Okamoto, R. (2014). Risk factors for the development of catheter-related bloodstream infections in patients receiving home parenteral nutrition. *Journal of Parenteral and Enteral Nutrition*, 38(6), 744–749.

Gorski, L. A., Hadaway, L., Hagle, M., McGoldrick, M., Orr, M., & Doellman, D. (2016). Infusion therapy standards of practice. *Journal of Infusion Nursing*, 39(1S), S1–S159.

Keller, S. C., Williams, D., Gavgani, M., Hirsch, D., Adamovich, J., Hohl, D., . . . Perl, T. M. (2016). Environmental exposures and the risk of central venous catheter complications and readmissions in home infusion therapy patients. *Infection Control and Hospital Epidemiology*, 38(1), 68–75.

McGoldrick, M. (2014). Bag technique: Preventing and controlling infections in home care and hospice. *Home Healthcare Now*, 32(1), 39–45.

McGoldrick, M. (2016). Core and supplementary contents in the home care nursing bag. *Home Healthcare Now*, 34(8), 457.

Mermel, L. A. (2011). What is the predominant source of intravascular catheter infections? *Clinical Infectious Diseases*, 52(2), 211–212.

Mutalib, M., Evans, V., Hughes, A., & Hill, S. (2015). Aseptic non-touch technique and catheter-related bloodstream infection in children receiving parenteral nutrition at home. *United European Gastroenterology Journal*, 3(4), 393–398.

O'Grady, N. P., Alexander, M., Burns L. A., Dellinger E. P., Garland J., Heard S.O., . . . Healthcare Infection Control Practices Advisory Committee. (2011). Guidelines for the prevention of intravascular catheter-related infections, 2011. Retrieved from http://www.cdc.gov/hicpac/pdf/guidelines/bsi-guidelines-2011.pdf

Phillips, L., & Gorski, L. A. (2014). *Manual of IV therapeutics: Evidence-based practice for infusion therapy.* Philadelphia, PA: F.A. Davis.

Rinke, M. L., Bundy, D. G., Milstone, A. M., Deuber, K., Chen, R., Colantuoni, E., & Miller, M. R. (2013). Bringing central line-associated bloodstream infection prevention home: CLABSI definitions and prevention policies in home health agencies. *The Joint Commission Journal on Quality and Safety, 39*(8), 361–370.

Rinke, M. L., Milstone, A. M., Chen, R., Mirski, K., Bundy, D. G., Colantuoni, E., . . . Miller, M. R. (2013). Ambulatory pediatric oncology CLABSIs: Epidemiology and risk factors. *Pediatric Blood Cancer, 60*(11), 1882–1889.

Rowley, S., Clare, S., Macqueen, S., & Molyneux, R. (2010). ANTT v2: An updated practice framework for aseptic technique. *British Journal of Nursing, 19*(5, Suppl.), S5–S11.

Safdar, N., Maki, D. G., & Mermel, L. A. (2014). Infections due to infusion therapy. In J. R. Jarvis (Ed.), *Bennett and Brachman's hospital infections* (6th ed., pp. 561–591). Philadelphia, PA: Lippincott Williams & Wilkins.

Shang, J., Larson, E., Liu, J., & Stone, P. (2015). Infection in home health care: Results from national Outcome and Assessment Information Set data. *American Journal of Infection Control, 43*(5), 454–459.

Shang, J., Ma, C., Poghosyan, L., Dowding, D., & Stone, P. (2014). The prevalence of infections and patient risk factors in home health care: A systematic review. *American Journal of Infection Control, 42*, 479–484.

Siegel, J. D., Rhinehart, E., Jackson, M., & Chiarello, L. (2007). Guideline for isolation precautions: Preventing transmission of infectious agents in healthcare settings. Retrieved from www.cdc.gov/ncidod/dhqp/hai.html

United Hospital Fund. (2016). Preventing central line-associated bloodstream infection (CLABSI) in the home setting: A toolkit. Retrieved from https://www.uhfnyc.org/publications/881133

Weber, D. J., Brown, V., Huslage, K., Sickber-Bennett, E., & Rutala, W. A. (2009). Device-related infections in home health care and hospice: Infection rates, 1998–2008. *Infection Control and Hospital Epidemiology, 30*(10), 1022–1024.

II

Access Devices
and Methods

4

Peripheral Catheters

Reliable vascular access is a major factor allowing for the success of home infusion therapy. Selecting the most appropriate vascular access device (VAD) as well as the site of placement is a critical decision that impacts the clinical outcome as well as the patient experience and satisfaction with care and this decision requires critical thinking and analysis of multiple factors (Gorski et al., 2016). Home infusion therapy via a peripheral catheter is less common than infusion via a central VAD (CVAD) due to the fact that many home infusion therapies involve irritating drugs or fluids and the duration of therapy is often weeks versus days.

Peripheral catheters include the traditional "short peripheral catheter," or SPC as referred to by the Infusion Nurses Society (INS), and midline catheters. Although use of the SPC is limited to shorter courses, the use of midline catheters for patients requiring a few weeks of infusion therapy is growing. This chapter provides an overview addressing appropriate use of peripheral catheters, care and maintenance guidelines, and potential complications.

After reading this chapter, the reader will be able to:

- Discuss indications for peripheral catheter placement
- Differentiate between short peripheral and midline catheters
- Describe catheter placement issues
- Identify potential complications of peripheral catheters

PATIENT SELECTION CONSIDERATIONS: PERIPHERAL VENOUS ACCESS

The patient is often referred to the home care agency with a VAD already in place. However, in some situations, the home care nurse is involved in the decision-making process. General guidance in selecting the most appropriate type of VAD is found in the INS standards under the VAD Planning Standard (Gorski et al., 2016, p. S51):

- Consider the prescribed therapy or treatment regimen; anticipated duration of therapy; vascular characteristics; and patient's age, comorbidities, history of infusion therapy, preference for VAD location, and ability and resources available to care for the device.
- VAD selection should be a collaborative process among the interprofessional team, the patient, and the patient's caregivers. With home care, patient preference should always be a consideration. For home infusion patients, consider safety and the impact on activities of daily living as well as ability to care for the VAD.
- The VAD selected should have the fewest number of lumens, have the smallest outer diameter, and be the least invasive device to meet the patient's needs. A peripheral catheter would be considered less invasive than a CVAD.

When considering a peripheral catheter, consider the anticipated duration of infusion therapy in conjunction with the prescribed infusate characteristics (irritant, vesicant, and high osmolarity) and the availability of peripheral sites.

- Duration of infusion therapy:
  - Consider the SPC when infusion therapy is anticipated for less than 1 week *if* the prescribed medication or solution is well tolerated by peripheral veins. An SPC is also an appropriate choice for patients who require infusions on a less frequent basis, such as the patient who requires an occasional dose of furosemide or infliximab infusions every 6 weeks.
  - Consider a midline catheter when infusion therapy is anticipated for more than 1 week and less than 3 to 4 weeks *if* the prescribed medication or solution is well tolerated by peripheral veins. Typical medications and solutions administered via a midline include antimicrobials, fluid replacement,

and analgesics. Caution is recommended with intermittent vesicant infusions due to the risk of undetected extravasation in the deep veins of the upper arm. Research on appropriate infusates via midline catheters continues to evolve.

- Avoid administration via peripheral catheters with continuous vesicant infusions, parenteral nutrition, or infusates with an osmolarity greater than 900 mOsm/L.

Fast Facts in a Nutshell

There are three layers of veins. The innermost layer of the vein is called the "tunica intima." It consists of a single, smooth layer of endothelial cells. These cells are easily damaged through a variety of insertion and/or care-related factors such as rapid catheter advancement, use of large catheters, catheter motion during dwell time due to lack of catheter stabilization, or poor insertion technique, allowing entry of microorganisms. Results of cellular damage include vein inflammation, infiltration, and infection. The "tunica media" is the middle layer of the vein, which is composed of muscular and elastic tissue and nerve fibers for vasoconstriction and vasodilation. The outermost vein layer is the "tunica adventitia," which consists of connective tissue that supports the vein. As part of the aging process, changes in venous structure can make placement of peripheral IV catheters challenging. The tunica intima, as well as the tunica media, become thicker making vein entry more difficult. Valves located within the veins also become more rigid and sclerotic (Coulter, 2016).

IDENTIFYING NONCYTOXIC VESICANTS

Cytotoxic vesicants used in cancer treatment are addressed in Chapter 11. The INS identified a "red" and "yellow" list of vesicants (Gorski et al., 2017). Red list vesicants, defined as well-recognized vesicants with multiple citations and reports of tissue damage upon extravasation, include dobutamine, dextrose solutions with greater than or equal to 12.5% dextrose concentration, parenteral nutrition solutions with an osmolarity greater than 900 mOsm/L. Yellow list vesicants are associated with fewer published reports of extravasation, but published drug information and infusate characteristics indicate caution and potential for tissue damage. Yellow list vesicants administered in home care include acyclovir, dextrose solutions with greater than or equal to 10.5% to 12.5% dextrose concentration, nafcillin, pentamidine, phenobarbital sodium, potassium greater than or equal to 60 mEq/L, and vancomycin.

TYPES OF PERIPHERAL IV CATHETERS

Short Peripheral IV Catheters

Description

- The SPC is approximately 2 inches or less in length. Choices of SPCs include stainless steel needles and the over-the-needle that leaves a plastic-type catheter in place. Stainless steel needles are indicated *only* for single-dose administration and are not left in place due to the increased risk of infiltration. Peripheral catheters with engineered safety devices are used.

Advantages

- Low risk of infection and catheter-related complications
- Low cost

Key Points Regarding Placement

- *Catheter Size:* Use smallest gauge catheter needed to deliver the infusion therapy; this allows for good blood flow around catheter decreasing the risk for phlebitis. A 22-gauge catheter is a common choice; a 24 gauge is also appropriate, especially for those with small, fragile veins including pediatric and older adult patients.

- *Site Selection:*
  - Select nondominant extremity whenever possible.
  - The forearm is recommended as it will likely last longer due to larger veins, have less movement (i.e., away from an area of flexion), be easier to stabilize, and have less interference with activities of daily living.
  - Consider activity level and patient needs before placing an SPC in the hand.
  - Avoid areas of flexion (e.g., antecubital fossa and wrist) and areas of previous venipuncture; subsequent peripheral intravenous (IV) insertions are always proximal or above previous sites.
  - Do not use lower extremities due to risk of tissue damage, thrombophlebitis, and ulceration.
  - Be aware of and avoid areas associated with increased risk for nerve damage: Cephalic vein at the wrist due to proximity to superficial radial nerve, palm side of the wrist due to proximity to median nerve, and antecubital fossa due to proximity to median/anterior interosseous/antebrachial nerves.
  - *Pediatric:* Veins of the scalp, and if not walking, the foot may be used. If the SPC is placed in the hand, avoid the hand where a child is thumb-sucking.
- *Vein Identification:*
  - A tourniquet is typically used. Loosely apply or avoid tourniquet use in patients who bruise easily, who are at risk for bleeding, have compromised circulation, and/or who have fragile veins (Gorski et al., 2016, p. S64).
  - Use of warmth, including dry heat, can be very successful in dilating veins.
  - Use of visualization technology: Ultrasound is increasingly used in acute care settings. There are also light devices that provide transillumination to identify veins. Another option is near infrared (nIR) light technology. Portable nIR units are available and are being used by some home care agencies. Deeper veins (e.g., 10 mm in depth) not visible to the naked eye may be identified by nIR. Specifically, bifurcations and valves may be identified and the venous pathway can be seen. For placement of SPCs in the forearm, nIR can be a valuable tool. As with any technology, the use of nIR requires specific education and training and competency assessment.

- *Aseptic Technique:*
  - Skin antisepsis is a critical step. Prior to skin antisepsis, if the skin is visibly dirty, cleanse with soap and water. If hair removal is indicated, use scissors and do not shave. The preferred antiseptic agent is >0.5% chlorhexidine in alcohol solution; if contraindicated, an iodophor, tincture of iodine, or 70% alcohol may be used. Apply for recommended time frame (e.g., 30 seconds) and allow to completely dry.
  - Use a new pair of disposable nonsterile gloves in conjunction with a no-touch technique—do not touch the insertion site after skin antisepsis.
- *Peripheral Attempts and Placement Issues:*
  - Use a 10 to 15 degree angle from the skin when inserting the SPC. For the older adult, use a lower angle of 5 to 15 degrees due to the loss of subcutaneous fat and more superficial veins. This will reduce the risk of going through the underside of the vein wall. Too often, the older adult patient endures multiple attempts at venous access (Coulter, 2016). Nurse knowledge and competency are essential for this prevalent home care population.
  - Make no more than two attempts at short peripheral catheter placement per clinician and limit total attempts to no more than four. It is important to recognize the consequences of multiple attempts at placement, which include pain, delayed treatment, limiting future vascular access, cost, and increased risk for complications. Patients with difficult vascular access require a careful assessment of VAD needs and collaboration with the health care team to discuss appropriate options (Gorski et al., 2016, p. S64). Although this is challenging to home care agencies, identifying and ensuring nurse competence in SPC placement is important to positive patient outcomes and patient satisfaction.
  - If nerve damage is suspected during the placement procedure based upon patient reporting of numbness, tingling, or other paresthesias, immediately remove the SPC and notify the physician (Gorski et al., 2016, p. S64). Early identification and intervention may reduce the risk of permanent nerve damage. Avoid probing for the vein as this increases the risk for nerve damage.
  - If an artery is inadvertently accessed, immediately remove and apply pressure to the site.

- *Catheter Stabilization:*
  - Purpose: To minimize the catheter movement at the hub, reducing the risk for dislodgement and other complications; the risk for mechanical phlebitis and infiltration is reduced when catheter movement is minimized.
  - An engineered stabilization device, specifically designed for stabilization, is preferred.

Fast Facts in a Nutshell

Safety-engineered devices, including SPCs, are used to reduce the risk for needlestick injury. The INS recommends the use of *passive* safety devices. Passive devices require no action on part of the user (while *active* safety devices require an action on the part of the user) to ensure that the needle or sharp is isolated after use (e.g., push a button). When using active safety devices, it is important that the nurse understand and properly activate the safety mechanism.

Midline Peripheral IV Catheters

Description

- The midline is a peripheral catheter defined by INS as a catheter inserted into the upper arm via the basilic, cephalic, or brachial vein, with the internal tip located at or near the level of the axilla and distal to the shoulder (Gorski et al., 2016, p. S152). Midline catheters are inserted only by nurses who have completed an education and competency program.

Advantages

- Low risk of infection and decreased risk of phlebitis
- Radiologic confirmation of tip placement not required
- Avoidance of frequent catheter replacement
- Expected dwell times are generally between 2 and 4 weeks; average dwell times have been reported: 13 days (Owen, 2014); 22 days (Sharp, Esterman, McCutcheon, Hearse, & Cummings, 2014); and in a retrospective study of 92 palliative home care patients, the median dwell time was 85 days and ranged from 1 to 365 days (Guiliani et al., 2013). No infectious complications were reported in these studies.

■ Decreased cost compared to a CVAD (Guiliani et al., 2013; Owen, 2014; Sharp et al., 2014).

Key Points Regarding Placement

■ *Avoid Midlines:* When there is a history of venous thrombosis, hypercoagulability, decreased venous flow to the extremities, or end-stage renal disease requiring peripheral vein preservation (Gorski et al., 2016, p. S52).

■ *Site Selection:*
  ▪ Select nondominant extremity whenever possible.
  ▪ Be aware of and avoid areas associated with increased risk for nerve damage: antecubital fossa due to proximity to median/anterior interosseous/antebrachial nerves.
  ▪ *Pediatric:* Additional site selections include veins in the leg with the catheter tip below groin level and the scalp with the catheter tip in the neck above the thorax.

■ *Vein Identification:*
  ▪ Use of visualization technology: Ultrasound is typically used to identify veins for midline catheter placement, which limits ability for placement in the home setting.

■ *Aseptic Technique:*
  ▪ Skin antisepsis is a critical step. The preferred agent is >0.5% chlorhexidine in alcohol solution; if contraindicated, an iodophor, tincture of iodine, or 70% alcohol may be used.
  ▪ Consider the use of maximal sterile barrier precautions with insertion (mask, gown, protective eyewear, cap, gloves, and large/full body drape). The use of a partial body drape may be as effective as a full body drape (Caparas, 2016).

COMPREHENSIVE CARE, ASSESSMENT, AND MONITORING

Regular Site Assessment (Figure 4.1)

■ With every home visit, assess for redness, tenderness, swelling, drainage, and/or the presence of paresthesias, numbness, or tingling at the site; the assessment includes visual assessment, palpation, and subjective information from the patient.

■ Assess midarm circumference prior to midline catheter placement or at first home visit to establish a baseline. Should there be a

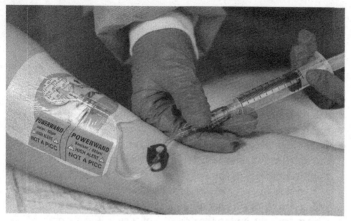

Figure 4.1 Powerwand midline catheter. *Source: Courtesy of Access Scientific, San Diego, CA.*

Note: Catheter site is properly stabilized and dressed. Note that dressing is labeled as "not a PICC." PICCs and midlines are generally inserted in the same veins and in the same area above the antecubital space. It is critically important for home care nurses to identify, document, and understand the implications for infusate administration based on the type of VAD.

suspicion of catheter-related venous thrombosis (pain, edema, erythema, and change in extremity mobility), remeasure midarm circumference to compare to baseline. In a prospective study of patients with peripherally inserted central catheters (PICC), a 3-cm or greater increase in arm circumference was associated with upper arm venous thrombosis (Maneval & Clemence, 2014). Although this study did not address midlines, there is also a risk of venous thrombosis with these catheters.

■ Assess and ensure catheter patency. Flush and aspirate for a blood return, defined as blood that has the color and consistency of whole blood, prior to each infusion. In the absence of a blood return, a decision *may* be made to infuse via the peripheral catheter based on the ability to freely flush the catheter, the absence of any patient complaints of discomfort with flushing, and the absence of any signs of infiltration or other complications. This decision must be made carefully. If the infusate is a vesicant, it should *not* be administered in the absence of a blood return.

Regular Site Care: Skin Antisepsis, Dressing Changes, Stabilization Devices

- Use aseptic technique.
- The preferred agent for routine skin antisepsis is >0.5% chlorhexidine in alcohol solution.
- Perform site care and dressing changes every 5 to 7 days when using a transparent semipermeable dressing (TSM); every 2 days if using a gauze dressing.
- Follow manufacturer's directions for placement and changing of the stabilization device. When using medical adhesive types of stabilization devices, be aware of the risk for medical adhesive–related skin injury (MARSI). The risk may be increased with very young and older patients due to fragility of skin, when there is joint movement, and in the presence of edema. The use of approved skin barrier solutions may reduce the risk. It is important to let the barrier solution fully dry before placement.
- Do not use rolled bandages, with or without elastic properties, to secure any type of VAD because they do not adequately secure the VAD, can obscure signs and symptoms of complications, and can impair circulation or the flow of infusion. The presence of skin disorders that contradict the use of medical adhesives (i.e., pediatric epidermolysis bullosa and toxic epidermal necrolysis) may necessitate the use of tubular gauze mesh rather than an adhesive-engineered stabilization device (Gorski et al., 2016, pp. S72–S74).

Flushing and Locking

- Purpose: VADs are flushed to assess and maintain patency and prevent precipitation due to incompatibilities between solutions or medications. Peripheral VADs are locked to maintain patency in between intermittent use.
- Use single-dose syringes for flushing and locking.
- Flush solution volume should be equal to or at least twice catheter volume capacity and any add-on devices.
- Lock solution volume should equal the internal volume of the VAD and any add-on devices plus 20%.
- Preservative-free saline (0.9% sodium chloride) is used to flush and lock SPCs. There is a lack of evidence for midline locking solutions; either saline (most common) or low concentration (10 U/mL) heparin is used.
- Lock peripheral catheters at least once per day.

- Use a syringe size in accordance with manufacturer's guidelines; many catheter manufacturers recommend use of a 10-mL barrel-sized syringe to reduce risk of catheter damage; 10-mL syringe use is an industry standard.
- Use a positive pressure technique to prevent reflux of blood into catheter (see the following).

Needleless Connectors (NCs)

- Disinfect prior to each access into the SPC or midline catheter. NCs are known sources of microbial contamination. Disinfection before the first access into the NC may not be necessary if the NC has been covered with a "passive disinfection cap" (see Chapter 3; Figure 3.2) that contains a disinfectant agent (typically alcohol); these caps are discarded after removal and a fresh cap placed after completion of the intermittent infusion. The INS suggests the use of a 5- to 15-second disinfectant scrub (e.g., 70% alcohol) prior to subsequent entries into the NC (Gorski et al., 2016).
- Know the type of NC used:
  - Positive displacement NCs push a small amount of fluid through the catheter lumen upon disconnection of the locking syringe → Implication: Do not clamp a catheter before disconnecting the syringe.
  - Neutral NCs have an internal mechanism that prevents blood reflux. Catheter clamping sequence does not impact NC function.
  - Negative displacement NCs allow blood reflux upon locking syringe disconnection → Implication: Clamp catheter as the syringe is disconnected.

Blood Withdrawal for Laboratory Sampling

- Blood can be withdrawn from SPCs based on analysis of risks versus benefits. It may be useful in pediatrics, adults with difficult venous access, and in presence of bleeding disorders. Risks include increased risk for infection due to catheter hub manipulation, loss of catheter patency, and erroneous laboratory values (Gorski et al., 2016, p. S87). There is a lack of data for recommending blood sampling off of midline catheters. The impact on catheter patency and accuracy of laboratory values is unknown.

Catheter Removal/Site Rotation: SPCs

- Remove the SPC or midline catheter as soon as it is no longer needed.
- Historically, the SPC was removed and replaced based on a period of time (e.g., every 96 hours). Based on research, the SPC may be left in place and removed and replaced based on clinical indications; for example, in the event of phlebitis or infiltration. There are no studies related to clinically indicated SPC removal and replacement in the home care setting. Critical issues that impact the dwell time of the SPC include appropriate site selection, appropriate device selection, and attention to conditions under which catheter is placed—aseptic technique is critical, SPC stabilization, and maintenance of intact dressing.

Monitoring for Complications

- See Table 4.1
- Reported and potential complications associated with midline catheters are relatively low/rare and include accidental dislodgements, phlebitis, infiltration, venous thrombosis, and infection (Caparas & Hu, 2014; Guiliani et al., 2013; Sharp et al., 2014; venous thrombosis is addressed in Chapter 5).

PATIENT EDUCATION: KEY POINTS

- Rationale for the peripheral catheter
- Advantages and disadvantages of alternative VADs
- Care and management requirements
- Infusate administration as appropriate (see Chapter 7)
- Potential risks/complications including signs and symptoms to report and how to report them
- Checking the SPC or midline catheter site for intactness of the dressing, and signs of complications at least daily. If a running peripheral infusion, instruct to check the site at least every 4 hours during waking hours (Gorski et al., 2016, p. S82)

CASE STUDY: PERIPHERAL IV SELECTION

Mr. Fox is a long-term home care patient with multiple diagnoses including multiple sclerosis with a neurogenic bladder, which has

Table 4.1

Potential Complications of Peripheral Catheters

Complication	Signs/symptoms	Prevention	Interventions
Infiltration/extravasation *Mechanical:* Catheter itself irritates or injures the endothelial cells lining the vein wall *Obstructive:* Blood clot formation and lymphedema *Pharmacologic or physiochemical properties associated with drug concentration/volume:* Extremes of pH, high osmolarity, and vasoconstrictors	■ Cool skin temperature at the site ■ Blanched/taut skin ■ Patient complaints of skin tightness, pain, or discomfort ■ Swelling ■ Decreased mobility of the extremity ■ Leaking of fluid from the insertion site ■ Changes in the infusion flow quality ■ Lack of a blood return	■ Appropriate infusate ■ Appropriate site ■ No more than two SPC attempts per nurse/four total ■ Small catheter ■ Never place new SPC below a previous site ■ Catheter stabilization ■ Do not rely on infusion pump as it will not detect upon infiltration	■ Stop infusion immediately ■ Vesicants: Attempt to aspirate any residual drug/IV fluid—do not flush! SPC removal—do not apply pressure ■ Limb elevation ■ Cold compresses to localize medication in the tissue and reduce inflammation (e.g., non-irritant and hyperosmolar fluids/medications) ■ Warm compresses to increase local blood flow and disperse medication through the tissue (e.g., vasopressors) ■ Document—measurement/description; estimated volume into tissue ■ Notify MD based on severity of infiltration/extravasation
Phlebitis Irritation of the vein intima provokes inflammation with	Phlebitis is graded according to INS Phlebitis Scale: 1—Erythema at site with or without pain	■ Appropriate infusate ■ Hand hygiene and aseptic technique with insertion and all IV procedures	■ Determine the potential etiology, whether chemical, mechanical, bacterial, or postinfusion phlebitis

(continued)

Table 4.1

Potential Complications of Peripheral Catheters (continued)

Complication	Signs/symptoms	Prevention	Interventions
fibrin deposition and thrombus formation. Causes: ■ Chemical (i.e., infusate related) ■ Mechanical (i.e., related to catheter movement) ■ Bacterial or infectious ■ Postinfusion (i.e., after SPC removal)	2—Pain at site with erythema and/or edema 3—Pain at site with erythema and/or edema, streak formation, and palpable venous cord 4—Pain at site with erythema and/or edema, streak formation, palpable venous cord > 1 inch in length, and purulent drainage (Gorski et al., 2016, p. S96)	■ Allow antiseptic to fully dry prior to catheter insertion and never touch skin after antisepsis ■ Small catheter ■ Avoid areas of flexion—if an area of flexion must be used, stabilize joint ■ Catheter stabilization	■ Remove the SPC and replace as clinically indicated ■ Monitor the site for postinfusion phlebitis for 48 hours ■ Treatment: Warm compress, elevate limb, analgesics as needed, and other pharmacologic interventions ■ Notify MD based on severity of phlebitis (e.g., grade 3 or 4)
Infection ■ Local site ■ Suppurative (purulent) thrombophlebitis: Serious peripheral-related infection—thrombus surrounding the cannula becomes infected leading to purulent drainage from the insertion site ■ Bloodstream infection	■ Local: Redness, swelling, induration, and/or drainage at the site ■ Bloodstream infection: Fever, chills, backache, nausea, malaise, headache, and hypotension	■ Hand hygiene before placement and before each access ■ Aseptic technique ■ Disinfect NC prior to catheter access	■ Notify physician ■ Remove catheter ■ Obtain cultures as ordered: Purulent drainage at site; catheter tip ■ Most often, catheter replacement ■ Sometimes, local infection treated ■ Topical as well as systemic antimicrobial treatment may be indicated

Nerve damage ■ Direct puncture nerve injury	■ Sharp shooting pain up or down the arm	■ Avoid sites at greater risk for nerve injury	■ Immediately remove catheter and notify the MD promptly—rapid attention may prevent permanent injury
■ Nerve compression injury may occur as a result of infiltration or extravasation of an infusion	■ Sensation of pain that changes in severity depending on needle position; "pins and needles" sensation or an "electric shock" feeling	*Dorsal hand*—distal sensory branches of the radial and ulnar nerves *Cephalic vein at the wrist*—superficial radial nerve	
	■ Pain or tingling in the hand or fingertips ■ Intensification of symptoms may be indicative of advancing nerve damage ■ Nerve compression injury due to severe infiltration/extravasation: Pain, pallor, paresthesias (e.g., numbness and tingling), paralysis, and/or pulselessness, restricted joint movement and resistance to passive motion	*Volar aspect of wrist*—median nerve *Antecubital fossa*—lateral and medial antebrachial nerves ■ Avoid subcutaneous probing for vein/multiple passes of needle ■ Control bleeding to reduce hematoma risk ■ Infiltration/extravasation prevention	

INS, Infusion Nurses Society; IV, intravenous; NC, needleless connectors; SPC, short peripheral catheter.

Sources: Phillips and Gorski (2014) and Alexander et al. (2014).

Chapter **4** Peripheral Catheters

resulted in placement of a suprapubic urinary catheter. He has signs and symptoms consistent with a urinary tract infection (UTI). A urine sample reveals an infection due to *Klebsiella pneumoniae*. Due to Mr. Fox's history of frequent UTIs and treatment, the culture sensitivities reveal resistance to several antibiotics but susceptible to the antibiotic cefapime. The MD has prescribed a 7-day course of every 12-hour cefapime via a peripheral catheter. Is a peripheral catheter appropriate? What if the infection required vancomycin treatment for the same period of time?

Discussion

Based on the duration of infusion therapy of 7 days, a peripheral catheter could be appropriate. Reviewing a reputable drug resource and discussion with the home infusion pharmacist, cefapime is not a vesicant and can be given peripherally. Furthermore, the nurse assesses Mr. Fox's veins, placing a blood pressure cuff on his arm to dilate the veins. His peripheral veins are adequate for cannulation. Mr. Fox understands that a peripheral IV will be placed for his antibiotics and that this is a good choice for him. Should the prescribed drug be vancomycin, the answer may be different. According to the INS, vancomycin is a "yellow" list vesicant and could cause tissue damage with extravasation. Continuous vesicant infusions are not appropriate for peripheral administration but vancomycin is usually administered intermittently. A few doses of vancomycin *could* be given peripherally if the patient's venous access is good and the catheter is placed in a large vein. Ongoing assessment is critical. Vancomycin may be administered via a midline catheter, although there is limited evidence for this practice and there is concern about the risk of extravasation in the deeper veins of the upper arm.

TEST YOUR KNOWLEDGE

1. Noncytotoxic vesicants that might be administered in the home include:
   a. Nafcillin
   b. Ceftriaxone
   c. Daptomycin
   d. Potassium 40 mEq/L
2. A common SPC catheter size is:
   a. 18 gauge
   b. 20 gauge

   c. 22 gauge

   d. 26 gauge

3. A recommended site for SPC placement is:

   a. The hand

   b. The forearm

   c. The antecubital space

   d. The wrist

4. nIR technology may be used to identify:

   a. Very deep veins 20 to 25 mm in depth

   b. Presence of venous valves

   c. Presence of a thrombus

   d. Nerve location

5. An advantage to the midline catheter is:

   a. Less frequent catheter replacements

   b. Less cost compared to an SPC

   c. An average dwell time of 4 to 6 weeks

   d. Decreased risk for venous thrombosis

6. The risk of MARSI is increased in:

   a. Patients who are obese

   b. Older patients

   c. Patients with midline catheters

   d. Patients with SPCs

7. When flushing via a positive displacement NC:

   a. Clamp the catheter before disconnecting the final locking syringe

   b. Clamp the catheter after disconnecting the final locking syringe

   c. The catheter clamping sequence does not matter

   d. Never clamp a catheter

8. A risk associated with blood sampling via an SPC includes:

   a. Phlebitis

   b. Infection

   c. Nerve damage

   d. Infiltration

ANSWERS

1. a

2. c

3. b

4. b

5. a
6. b
7. b
8. b

References

Alexander, M., Gorski, L. A., Corrigan, A., Bullock, M., Dickenson, A., & Earhart, A. (2014). Technical and clinical application. In M. Alexander, A. Corrigan, L. A. Gorski, & L. Phillips (Eds.), *Core curriculum for infusion nursing* (5th ed., pp. 1–85). Philadelphia, PA: Lippincott Williams & Wilkins.

Caparas, J. V. (2016). Maximal sterile barrier versus partial-body drape for midline insertion. Poster presentation. Presented at the Association of Vascular Access Annual Scientific Meeting, Orlando, FL.

Caparas, J. V., & Hu, J. (2014). Safe administration of vancomycin through a novel midline catheter: A randomized, prospective clinical trial. *Journal of Vascular Access*, 15(4), 251–256.

Coulter, K. (2016). Successful infusion therapy in older adults. *Journal of Infusion Nursing*, 39(6), 352–358.

Gorski, L. A., Hadaway, L., Hagle, M., McGoldrick, M., Orr, M., & Doellman, D. (2016). Infusion therapy standards of practice. *Journal of Infusion Nursing*, 39(1S), S1–S159.

Gorski, L. A., Stranz, M., Cook, L., Joseph, J. M., Kokotis, K., Sabatino-Holmes, P., & VanGosen, L. (2017). Development of an evidence-based list of noncytotoxic vesicant medications and solutions. *Journal of Infusion Nursing*, 40(1), 26–40.

Krzywda, E., & Meyer, D. (2014). Parenteral nutrition. In M. Alexander, A. Corrigan, L. A. Gorski, & L. Phillips (Eds.), *Core curriculum for infusion nursing* (5th ed., pp. 309–355). Philadelphia, PA: Lippincott Williams & Wilkins.

Guiliani, J., Andreeta, L., Mattiola, M., Melotto, A., Zuliani, S., Zanardi, O., & Borese, B. (2013). Intravenous midline catheter usage: Which clinical impact in homecare patients? *Journal of Palliative Care Medicine*, 16(6), 598.

Maneval, R. E., & Clemence, B. J. (2014). Risk factors associated with catheter-related upper extremity deep vein thrombosis in patients with peripherally inserted central venous catheters. *Journal of Infusion Nursing*, 37(4), 260–268.

Owen, K. (2014). The use of 8 cm midlines in community IV therapy. *British Journal of Nursing* 23(Suppl.), S18–S20.

Phillips, L., & Gorski, L. A. (2014). *Manual of IV therapeutics: Evidence-based practice for infusion therapy*. Philadelphia, PA: F.A. Davis.

Sharp, R., Esterman, A., McCutcheon, H., Hearse, N., & Cummings, M. (2014). The safety and efficacy of midlines compared to peripherally inserted central catheters for adult cystic fibrosis patients: A retrospective, observational study. *International Journal of Nursing Studies*, 51, 694–702.

5

Central Vascular Access Devices

As discussed in the Chapter 4, reliable vascular access is a critical factor in successful home infusion therapy. Central vascular access devices (CVADs), commonly called "central lines," are often placed for home infusion therapy because many home infusion therapies involve irritating drugs or fluids that would not be appropriate for peripheral infusion, or the anticipated duration of therapy is weeks to months. There are four main types of CVADs that are described in this chapter. Regardless of the type of CVAD, a central line is defined based on the internal location of the catheter tip. The tip should be located in the lower segment of the superior vena cava at or near the cavoatrial junction (Gorski, Hadaway, Hagle, McGoldrick, Orr, & Doellman, 2016).

This chapter provides a description of the four types of CVADs, care and maintenance guidelines, and potential complications.

After reading this chapter, the reader will be able to:

- Differentiate between the four types of CVADs
- Describe indications for CVADs
- Summarize major aspects of CVAD care and maintenance
- Identify potential complications of CVADs

PATIENT SELECTION CONSIDERATIONS: CENTRAL VASCULAR ACCESS

The patient who requires a CVAD is most often referred to the home care agency with the CVAD already in place. In some situations, the home care nurse is involved in the decision-making process. If the patient's infusion therapy is not appropriate for peripheral administration, as addressed in the previous chapter, a central line may be appropriate. Any type of infusion therapy may be administered via a central line. When selecting the type of central line, the process is collaborative among the interprofessional team, the patient, and the patient's caregivers. For home infusion patients, consider the safety and the impact on activities of daily living as well as ability to care for the VAD. A qualitative study aimed at understanding the patient experience of peripherally inserted central catheters (PICCs) examined the experience of living with a VAD (Sharp et al., 2014). Themes identified included apprehension/adaptation/acceptance, impact of treatment, asking questions, and freedom (to receive treatment at home). Of note, although INS standards (Gorski, Hadaway, Hagle, McGoldrick, Meyer, & Orr, 2016) recommended the use of sites in the nondominant arm, arm choice had a marginal impact on activities of daily living for these study participants. The researchers asserted the importance of involving patients in clinical decision making by providing them individualized education and support needed as they adapt to living with the PICC.

The catheter with the fewest number of lumens to meet the patient's needs is selected. When there are fewer lumens, there is less manipulation and access to the central circulation, which decreases the risk for catheter-related bloodstream infection. Furthermore, care is simplified for the patient.

TYPES OF CVADs

Peripherally Inserted Central Catheters

Description

- The PICC is a central line that is inserted into the veins in the region above the antecubital fossa—the cephalic, basilic, or median cubital. PICCs are placed at the bedside by infusion team nurses who have completed education, training, and competency requirements as defined by the health care organization. PICCs are placed also by physicians or competent nurses in the radiology suite. Less commonly, PICCs are placed in the home by special nurse teams that utilize ultrasound and have radiology services available for catheter tip placement verification. PICCs, like all central lines, are placed under the conditions of maximal sterile barrier precautions with an independent observer ensuring that technique is not breached during catheter placement. It is important to recognize that PICCs are associated with an appreciable risk for catheter-associated vein thrombosis, especially in higher risk populations such as those patients with a cancer diagnosis. To reduce this risk, the catheter-to-vein ratio should be equal to or less than 45%, which allows more blood flow around the catheter in the vein (Gorski, Hadaway, Hagle, McGoldrick, Orr, & Doellman, 2016).

Advantages

- Outside of the acute care setting, a low risk of infection
- More reliable venous access than peripheral catheters
- Lower cost of placement when compared to subcutaneously tunneled catheters/implanted vascular access ports
- Single-, double-, and triple-lumen catheters available; most home infusion patients require only a single lumen
- Can be used for routine blood draws
- Can be removed in the home

Indications

- Expected duration of intravenous (IV) therapy lasting for weeks, and generally up to a year. However, any CVAD is not removed based on dwell time because there is no known optimal dwell time (Gorski, Hadaway, Hagle, McGoldrick, Orr, & Doellman, 2016). In other words, if the PICC is functioning well without any signs of complications, it can continue to be used.
- Patients requiring any moderate- to long-term infusion therapy such as antimicrobial drugs, chemotherapy, and parenteral nutrition.

Subcutaneously Tunneled Central Catheters

Description

- The subcutaneously tunneled catheter is a surgically placed central line. The catheter is tunneled underneath the skin,

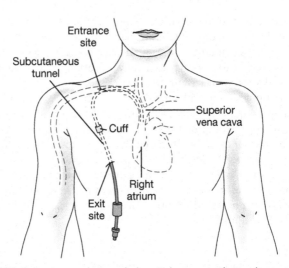

Figure 5.1 Subcutaneously tunneled central venous catheter placement.

Note: Note the catheter entrance site, where it enters the venous circulation, often via the internal jugular or subclavian vein, and the exit site, which is the focus of catheter site care.

usually on the chest wall. The catheter "entrance site" is located in the area of the clavicle where there is a small closed incision; this is the area where the catheter enters the venous circulation (Figure 5.1). The catheter is tunneled to an "exit site" lower on the chest where the catheter extrudes from the skin. A small synthetic "cuff" attached to the catheter is located within the subcutaneous tunnel and over time, the tissue attaches to the cuff and stabilizes the catheter in place (Figure 5.2). After the site is well healed, the catheter is difficult to dislodge and may even be managed without a dressing (Gorski, Hadaway, Hagle, McGoldrick, Orr, & Doellman, 2016). These catheters are often generically referred to as Hickman or Broviac catheters, although these are registered trademark names for catheters made by Bard Access Systems.

Advantages

- Long-term catheter with relatively low risk of infection and catheter-related complications
- Repairable
- Single-, double-, and triple-lumen catheters available

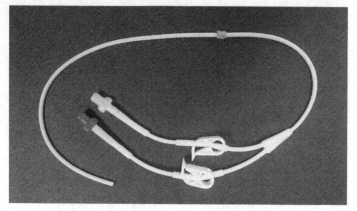

Figure 5.2 Subcutaneously tunneled catheter.
Note: Note the synthetic "cuff" that is attached to the catheter.

- Can be used for routine blood draws
- May remain in place for months to years
- May not require dressing after tunnel tract is well healed

Indications

- Expected duration of IV therapy months to years
- Patients requiring long-term parenteral nutrition, chemotherapy, or other long-term infusions

Nontunneled Central Vascular Catheters

Description

- Refers to the percutaneously placed catheter that may be placed via the subclavian or internal jugular route. These catheters are placed by a physician or competent infusion team nurse in the acute care setting. They are infrequently used in home care, but some patients may be discharged with a nontunneled catheter in place to complete shorter courses of home infusion therapy.

Advantages

- Lower cost of insertion compared to subcutaneously tunneled catheters
- Single-, double-, triple-, and quadruple-lumen catheters available

- Can be used for routine blood draws
- May be removed in the home setting; however, there is appreciable risk of air embolism during removal

Indications

- Expected duration of IV therapy days to weeks
- Any infusion therapy requiring central vascular access

Implanted Vascular Access Ports

Description

- The implanted vascular access port is a surgically placed device. Patients may have ports placed in outpatient surgery by a surgeon or, alternatively, they may be placed by an interventional radiologist in the radiology department. Placed completely underneath the skin, the port consists of a catheter attached to a reservoir (port) and is accessed through the skin using a special noncoring (i.e., Huber) needle. The port may be located in the chest (Figure 5.3), but there are also peripheral ports where the port body is located in the antecubital area (the catheter is threaded through the peripheral veins to the superior vena cava, like a PICC).

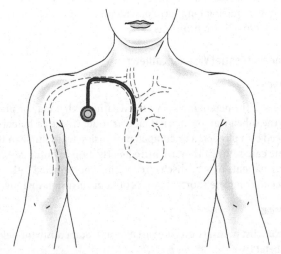

Figure 5.3 Implanted venous access port placement in the chest.

Advantages

- Low risk of infection and catheter-related complications
- Improved body image—no external evidence of port other than a small "bump"
- Single- and double-lumen catheters available
- Can be used for routine blood draws
- Minimal maintenance required—no dressing unless being actively used for infusion; usually monthly catheter locking (heparin or saline) to maintain patency
- May remain in place for months to years

Indications

- Expected duration of IV therapy months to years
- Patients with intermittent need for infusion therapy (e.g., chemotherapy and transfusions)
- Patients on long-term cyclic parenteral nutrition who prefer to access the port for every infusion than live with an external device

COMPREHENSIVE CARE, ASSESSMENT, AND MONITORING

Regular Site Assessment

- With every home visit, assess for intactness of the dressing, presence of any site redness, tenderness, swelling, drainage, and/or the presence of paresthesias, numbness, or tingling at the site; evidence of possible CVAD-associated venous thrombosis including edema/pain/engorged peripheral veins in the extremity, and/or difficulty with neck/extremity motion. The assessment includes visual assessment, palpation, and subjective information from the patient.
- Measure external catheter length at each visit and compare to previous measurements to identify possible catheter dislodgement.
- Assess midarm circumference prior to PICC placement or at first home visit to establish a baseline (Gorski, Hadaway, Hagle, McGoldrick, Orr, & Doellman, 2016, p. S29). Should there be a suspicion of catheter-related venous thrombosis (pain, edema, erythema, and change in extremity mobility), remeasure midarm circumference to compare to baseline. In a prospective study of patients with peripherally inserted central catheters (PICC), a 3-cm or greater increase in arm circumference was associated with upper arm venous thrombosis (Maneval & Clemence, 2014).

■ Assess and ensure catheter patency. Flush and aspirate for a
blood return, defined as blood that has the color and consistency
of whole blood (Gorski, Hadaway, Hagle, McGoldrick, Orr, &
Doellman, 2016) prior to each infusion.

Fast Facts in a Nutshell

Should the patient be taught to aspirate for a blood return prior to
each use? Although there is no clear guidance or consensus regarding this practice, this author believes that most patients should not
be instructed in this aspect of the procedure as it involves more
catheter manipulation and may increase the risk of occlusion.
Rather instruct the patient to immediately report any difficulties
with catheter flushing such as resistance or pain. If present, instruct
to notify the home care nurse for further assessment. Exceptions
may include the patient who is completely independent with long-
term or life-long infusion therapy.

Regular Site Care: Skin Antisepsis, Dressing Changes, and Stabilization Devices

■ Use aseptic technique.
■ The preferred agent for skin antisepsis is >0.5% chlorhexidine in
alcohol solution.
■ Perform site care and dressing changes every 5 to 7 days when
using a transparent semipermeable dressing (TSM); every 2 days
if using a gauze dressing or as needed if dressing is not intact, or
there is presence of drainage under the dressing. Failure to do so
increases the risk for infection due to the growth of microorganisms on the skin.
■ Follow manufacturer's directions for placement and changing of
the stabilization device. When using medical adhesive types of
stabilization devices, be aware of the risk for medical adhesive–
related skin injury (MARSI). The risk may be increased with very
young and older patients due to fragility of skin, when there is
joint movement, and in the presence of edema. The use of
approved skin barrier solutions may reduce the risk. It is
important to let the barrier solution fully dry before placement.
■ Do not use rolled bandages, with or without elastic properties, to
secure the PICC because they do not adequately secure, can

obscure signs and symptoms of complications, and can impair circulation or the flow of infusion. The presence of skin disorders that contradict the use of medical adhesives (i.e., pediatric epidermolysis bullosa and toxic epidermal necrolysis) may necessitate the use of tubular gauze mesh rather than adhesive-engineered stabilization device (Gorski, Hadaway, Hagle, McGoldrick, Orr, & Doellman, 2016, pp. S72–S74).

Implanted Port Access

- Use only noncoring safety needles; a recoil action when removing the port needle can result in an inadvertent clinician needlestick injury unless using a safety product (International Sharps Injury Prevention Society [ISIPS], 2016).
- Use the smallest gauge needle (e.g., 22 gauge) to prolong port life and reduce pain during insertion.
- Choose a needle length that allows it to sit flush to the skin and securely within the port to reduce the risk of needle dislodgement during infusion; a common length is 0.75 inch; shorter (0.5 inch) or longer (1–1.5 inches) may be needed based on the depth of the port.
- For continuous infusions via the port, change the noncoring needle/infusion system at least every 7 days.
- Consider the use of an anesthetic based on patient's pain tolerance and preferences; simple ice can be used; anesthetic creams (lidocaine/prilocaine) are effective but must remain on the skin for 45 to 60 minutes before port access. Distraction and relaxation techniques may also be effective.
- Use aseptic technique including sterile gloves and a mask during port access.

Fast Facts in a Nutshell

Aseptic technique and skin antisepsis are critically important when accessing the implanted port. When aseptic technique is compromised or when skin antisepsis is inadequate, microbes residing on the skin are tracked into the port, gaining access to the circulation and increasing the risk of a bloodstream infection (BSI). Competency assessment and validation should be a requirement for nurses who access ports.

Flushing and Locking

- Purpose: Flush the CVAD to assess and maintain patency and prevent precipitation due to incompatibilities between solutions or medications. Lock the CVAD to maintain patency in between use.
- Use single-dose syringes for flushing and locking.
- Flush solution volume should be equal to or at least twice catheter volume capacity and any add-on devices.
- Lock solution volume should equal the internal volume of the CVAD and any add-on devices plus 20%.
- Use preservative-free saline (0.9% sodium chloride) to flush central lines; use either saline or low concentration heparin (10 U/mL) to lock the central line; the use of heparin is considered for PICCs in home care due to reduced occlusion problems (Gorski, Hadaway, Hagle, McGoldrick, Orr, & Doellman, 2016, p. S78; Lyons & Phalen, 2014).
- Antimicrobial solutions (e.g., ethanol, citrate, and supratherapeutic antibiotic concentrations) may be used for catheter locking in patients with long-term CVADs, or patients with a history of frequent catheter-related BSIs (CR-BSIs). Ethanol is not recommended for catheters made of polyurethane material.
- Use a syringe size in accordance with manufacturer's guidelines; most catheter manufacturers recommend use of a 10-mL syringe to reduce risk of catheter damage; 10-mL syringe use is an industry standard.
- Use a positive pressure technique to prevent reflux of blood into catheter (see the following).

Fast Facts in a Nutshell

Always aspirate an antimicrobial lock solution at the end of the locking period. The solution is not flushed into the patient's bloodstream due to the risk of antibiotic resistance or other adverse effects (Gorski, Hadaway, Hagle, McGoldrick, Orr, & Doellman, 2016).

Needleless Connectors (NCs)

- Disinfect (using 70% alcohol, iodophors, or chlorhexidine in alcohol solution) prior to any catheter access using a vigorous mechanical scrub and allow to dry. NCs are known sources of microbial contamination.

- Disinfection caps: These are plastic caps that contain an antiseptic solution and are placed on the NC in between intermittent infusions; caps protect disinfection between intermittent use of CVADs. After removal of the cap for catheter access (i.e., flushing and tubing connection), the NC does not need to be disinfected; for subsequent NC access, the INS recommends consideration of disinfection as previously mentioned using a vigorous mechanical scrub.
- Understand the type of NC used: Positive displacement NCs push a small amount of fluid through the catheter lumen upon disconnection of the locking syringe (never clamp before disconnecting the syringe). Neutral NCs have an internal mechanism that prevents blood reflux, thus catheter clamping sequence does not impact NC function. Negative displacement NCs allow blood reflux upon locking syringe disconnection; clamping as the syringe is disconnected is recommended.
- Change the NC no more often than every 96 hours, or after blood culture sample, and upon contamination. In home care, the NC is often changed every 7 days at the time of the site care and dressing change.

Blood Withdrawal for Laboratory Sampling

- Blood can be withdrawn from CVADs based on analysis of risks versus benefits. Risks include infection due to catheter hub manipulation, loss of catheter patency, and erroneous laboratory values (Gorski, Hadaway, Hagle, McGoldrick, Orr, & Doellman, 2016, p. S87).
- For patients receiving parenteral nutrition, blood sampling from the CVAD is not recommended due to increased risk for CR-BSI (Ayers et al., 2014; Buchman, Opilla, Kwasny, Diamantidis, & Okamoto, 2014).

Monitoring for Complications

- As discussed in Chapter 3, infection may be less common in home care as compared to the acute care setting, but certain populations are at higher risk, such as those patients receiving parenteral nutrition, pediatric patients, and those who are immunocompromised. Regardless, infections are considered a preventable complication. Catheter occlusion secondary to thrombotic or precipitate is a more common complication that may be reduced with sound flushing and locking techniques. In Table 5.1, these complications as well as air embolism, catheter damage and malposition, venous thrombosis, and infiltration/extravasation are presented including signs/symptoms, prevention, and interventions.

PATIENT EDUCATION: KEY POINTS

- Check the CVAD site and dressing daily
- What to report:
  - Signs and symptoms to report include site or extremity redness/pain, swelling, hardness; fever, chills, difficulty in flushing/inability to flush, any unusual symptoms
  - Dressing not intact or drainage/blood present under dressing
- How to and whom to report symptoms
- Hand hygiene, aseptic technique, and disinfection of NCs
- Site protection; keeping VAD dressing/tubing dry during bathing; using a designated product or plastic wrap (see Figure 3.3 in Chapter 3)
- Implanted ports: Making sure women's bra straps or car seat belts do not irritate the accessed port; how to stop infusion if any wetness, leaking, or swelling at port site
- Never disconnect or reconnect administration set or NCs from catheter hub unless instructed to do so
- Ensure availability of a clamp/hemostat to use in event of ruptured/damaged CVAD and instruct in how to use
- Never forcibly flush or administer any infusion
- Never use scissors or any type of cutting tool near the CVAD

CASE STUDY: IMPLANTED PORT MALPOSITION

Mr. Deer has had an implanted port for over a year, which is used for infusing chemotherapy and periodic hydration fluids. It was functioning well for over a year, infusing without problems, and yielding a blood return upon aspiration. Now the home care nurse is unable to obtain a blood return and notes it does not flush as easily. The patient reported that he had an unusually intense period of coughing a few days earlier. The port problems were reported and the physician ordered alteplase. Despite repeated alteplase use on the advice of the physician, the problem continued. With each attempt at port access,

Table 5.1

Potential CVAD Complications

Complication	Signs/symptoms	Prevention	Interventions
Air embolism	■ Sudden onset dyspnea, coughing, chest pain, hypotension, wheezing, tachypnea ■ A loud continuous churning sound over precordium during auscultation	■ Prime all IV tubing/add-on devices ■ Clamp CVAD when disconnecting IV tubing/NC ■ Never use scissors near CVAD ■ During catheter removal, position patient in supine position removal, Valsalva maneuver, occlusive dressing upon removal	■ Take immediate action ■ Locate source of air entry and resolve ■ Place patient on left lateral decubitus position with head down ■ Initiate basic life support as needed, call 911
Catheter damage	■ Crack or hole in catheter ■ Could progress to signs/symptoms of air embolism if not immediately addressed	■ Never forcefully flush against resistance ■ Never use scissors near CVAD	■ Take immediate action to clamp between insertion site and damaged CVAD ■ Collaborate with health care team to discuss risks vs. benefits prior to CVAD repair ■ CVAD removal and replacement as appropriate

(continued)

Table 5.1

Potential CVAD Complications *(continued)*

Complication	Signs/symptoms	Prevention	Interventions
CVAD malposition *Primary malposition* occurs at the time of placement; this complication is not addressed here *Secondary malposition* is also called tip migration. Tip migration can occur at any time during the catheter dwell time	■ Absence of blood return ■ Changes in color/pulsatility of blood return ■ Difficulty in flushing ■ Shoulder, neck, chest pain or edema ■ Hearing a gurgling sound during flushing on side of CVAD ■ Palpitations	■ Not necessarily preventable except to stabilize CVAD to prevent outward CVAD migration	■ Report signs/symptoms ■ Never advance any external portion of the CVAD back into the insertion site ■ Do not infuse through a malpositioned CVAD until tip position established ■ Anticipate diagnostic testing such as chest x-ray with/without contrast injection ■ Provide physician/radiology department with clinical information so proper evaluation of CVAD can be done
CVAD occlusion Causes include mechanical problems, precipitate, or thrombotic	■ Inability to flush CVAD ■ Sluggish flow ■ Inability to aspirate blood ■ Frequent occlusion alarms on electronic infusion device	■ Proper flushing and locking ■ Appropriate clamping sequence based on type of NC ■ Do not allow infusion containers to run dry	■ Rule out mechanical causes such as clamps and kinked tubing ■ Rule out catheter malposition (see CVAD malposition); sometimes repositioning or bodily movement may result in ability to flush and obtain blood return. For ongoing/persistant problems, see CVAD malposition

CVAD-associated venous thrombosis

Contributing factors to venous thrombosis based on Virchow's triad:

- Hypercoagulability (e.g., common in patients with cancer diagnosis)
- Venous stasis (presence of CVAD slows blood flow within vein)
- Vein damage

- Pain/swelling in extremity, shoulder, neck, and chest
- Engorged peripheral veins
- Difficulty with neck/extremity motion
- Could progress to signs/symptoms of pulmonary embolism (e.g., dyspnea, pleuritic pain, diaphoresis, anxiety)

- Not always preventable
- Use smaller catheters to allow better blood flow (catheter-to-vein ratio 45% or less)
- Ensure optimal tip location
- Nonpharmacologic prevention strategies may include mobilization and use of extremity with PICC, performing normal activities of daily living, hydration

- Nonthrombotic causes such as precipitate or lipid build-up from 3-in-1 parenteral nutrition solutions may be cleared with agents such as hydrochloric acid, sodium bicarbonate, 70% ethanol (usually outpatient—must have policies in place)
- Thrombotic causes may be treated with thrombolytic agent (e.g., alteplase); this may be done in the home setting by competent nurses when policies in place
- Report signs/symptoms
- Anticipate diagnostic testing such as Doppler ultrasound in veins of upper extremity or venography with contrast injection
- Provide physician/radiology department with clinical information so proper evaluation of CVAD can be done
- Anticipate treatment with anticoagulants; usually CVAD not removed unless no longer needed for infusion therapy

(continued)

Chapter **5** Central Vascular Access Devices

Table 5.1

Potential CVAD Complications *(continued)*

Complication	Signs/symptoms	Prevention	Interventions
Infection	■ Local site: Redness, swelling, induration, and/or drainage ■ Port pocket: Erythema, tenderness, induration, exudate, surgical wound dehiscence, altered skin integrity over port ■ Subcutaneous tract: Erythema, induration, tenderness ■ Bloodstream infection: Fever, chills, backache, nausea, malaise, headache, hypotension	■ Hand hygiene before placement and before each access ■ Aseptic technique during all infusion-related procedures ■ Site protection during bathing and showering ■ Disinfect NC prior to catheter access ■ CVAD removal when no longer needed; obtain order to remove or refer to MD office/ outpatient	■ Notify physician ■ Based on severity of symptoms, hospitalization often warranted ■ Monitor VAD site, vital signs, laboratory findings, response to interventions ■ Replace administration set ■ Obtain cultures as ordered: Purulent drainage at site; blood cultures ■ Systemic antimicrobial treatment

Infiltration/extravasation	Lack of a blood return	Select a needle length adequate to pierce implanted vascular access port septum and contact base of the port	Stop infusion immediately
Causes associated with CVADs include: ■ Incomplete port needle insertion ■ Separation of catheter from port body ■ Loss of catheter integrity (e.g., hole/crack in catheter) ■ Catheter tip migration ■ Backtracking of drug along the tunnel resulting from fibrin sheath development	■ Leaking of fluid from the insertion site ■ Changes in the infusion flow quality ■ Resistance during fluid administration (e.g., during VAD flushing, electronic infusion device occlusion alarms) ■ Complaints of pain, tightness, burning, discomfort at, or around the insertion site, catheter tip, or entire venous pathway ■ Raised area on neck or chest	■ Stabilize noncoring needle of implanted vascular access port to reduce risk of dislodgement ■ Prior to infusion initiation and during infusion, assess CVAD for integrity, for a blood return, and absence of resistance to flushing	■ Vesicants: Attempt to aspirate any residual drug/IV fluid—do not flush! ■ Document including measurement and description of site; estimated volume into tissue ■ Notify MD

Phlebitis

Refer to Table 4.1.

Early mechanical phlebitis may occur shortly (first few days) after PICC placement and may be treated with compresses and arm elevation; when signs of phlebitis occur later, PICC removal is usually warranted.

CVAD, central vascular access device; IV, intravenous; NC, needleless connector; PICC, peripherally inserted central catheter; VAD, vascular access device.

Sources: Gorski, Hadaway, Hagle, McGoldrick, Meyer, & Orr (2016); Gorski, Hadaway, Hagle, McGoldrick, Orr, & Doellman (2016).

difficulty in obtaining a blood return continued unless the alteplase was used. Finally, the nurse stated that she did not feel comfortable administering more alteplase. She suggested that maybe there is a change in the catheter tip position or a more significant thrombotic problem and that this patient might benefit from radiological evaluation of the port. The physician agreed and under fluoroscopy, the radiologist found that the right subclavian–placed implanted port had its catheter projecting superiorly looped into the right internal jugular vein, and therefore was malpositioned. The catheter was able to be repositioned by the interventional radiologist.

Discussion

Malposition of CVADs is a potential problem during catheter dwell time. Referred to as "secondary malposition" or "tip migration," it can occur at any time during the catheter dwell time. Inability to obtain a blood return in the absence of other signs or symptoms is often a sign of a thrombotic problem such as a fibrin tail at the tip of the catheter. Although this was not an inappropriate first intervention, the need for repeated use does suggest other potential problems. Referring to Table 5.1, tip migration signs and symptoms include an absence of blood return, changes in color/pulsatility of blood return, and difficulty in flushing. The intense coughing episode was a possible contributing factor to the malposition. Suboptimal tip position may increase the risk of venous thrombosis. It was appropriate for the home care nurse to suggest the need for diagnostic testing. The highly educated and competent home care nurse assesses and recognizes potential CVAD complications and collaborates with the health care team to provide appropriate interventions.

TEST YOUR KNOWLEDGE

1. The internal location of the CVAD tip should be:
   a. Mid superior vena cava
   b. The right atrium
   c. Lower superior vena cava
   d. The subclavian vein
2. An increase in midarm circumference may be a sign of:
   a. Catheter malposition
   b. Venous thrombosis
   c. Infection
   d. Catheter occlusion

3. Blood sampling for laboratory testing is not recommended for:
   a. Patients with implanted ports
   b. Pediatric patients
   c. Patients receiving parenteral nutrition
   d. Patients with PICCs
4. Of the following, the most appropriate indication for placement of a subcutaneously tunneled catheter would be:
   a. Six weeks of IV antibiotic therapy
   b. Parenteral nutrition administration
   c. Fluid replacement for dehydration
   d. Intermittent chemotherapy infusions
5. An antimicrobial solution that may be used for catheter locking is:
   a. Ethanol
   b. Low concentration antibiotic solutions
   c. Heparin
   d. Alteplase
6. The risk of air embolism is reduced during catheter removal when the following step is taken:
   a. Position patient in the semi-Fowler's position during removal
   b. Place a gauze dressing over the site after removal
   c. Place patient in supine position during removal
   d. Have patient take a deep breath during removal
7. A factor that contributes to the risk of venous thrombosis includes:
   a. Engorged peripheral veins
   b. Suboptimal catheter tip position
   c. Presence of a precipitate
   d. A crack in the catheter
8. The risk of CVAD occlusion may be reduced by:
   a. Site protection during bathing
   b. Placement of smaller catheters
   c. Saline flushing between medication infusions
   d. Use of occlusive dressings.

ANSWERS

1. c
2. b
3. c
4. b

5. a
6. c
7. b
8. c

References

Ayers, P., Adams, S., Boullata, J., Gervasio, J., Holcombe, B., Kraft, M. D., . . . Worthington, P. (2014). A.S.P.E.N. parenteral nutrition safety consensus recommendations. *Journal of Parenteral and Enteral Nutrition, 38*(3), 291–333.

Buchman, A. L., Opilla, M., Kwasny, M., Diamantidis, T. G., & Okamoto, R. (2014). Risk factors for the development of catheter-related bloodstream infections in patients receiving home parenteral nutrition. *Journal of Parenteral and Enteral Nutrition, 38*(6), 744–749.

Gorski, L. A., Hadaway, L., Hagle, M., McGoldrick, M., Meyer, B., & Orr, M. (2016). *Policies and procedures for infusion therapy.* Norwood, MA: Infusion Nurses Society.

Gorski, L. A., Hadaway, L., Hagle, M., McGoldrick, M., Orr, M., & Doellman, D. (2016). Infusion therapy standards of practice. *Journal of Infusion Nursing, 39*(1S), S1–S159.

International Sharps Safety Prevention Society. (2016). Safety Huber needle. Retrieved from http://www.isips.org/page/safety_products/safety_huber_needle

Lyons, M. G., & Phalen, A. G. (2014). A randomized controlled comparison of flushing protocols in home care patients with peripherally inserted central catheters. *Journal of Infusion Nursing, 37*(4), 270–281.

Maneval, R. E., & Clemence, B. J. (2014). Risk factors associated with catheter-related upper extremity deep vein thrombosis in patients with peripherally inserted central venous catheters. *Journal of Infusion Nursing, 37*(4), 260–268.

Sharp, R., Grech, C., Fielder, A., Mikocka-Walus, A., Cummings, M., & Esterman, A. (2014). The patient experience of a peripherally inserted central catheter (PICC): A qualitative descriptive study. *Contemporary Nurse, 48*(1), 26–35.

6

Other Infusion Access Methods

Although intravenous (IV) infusion of medications and fluids is the most common type of home infusion therapy, the home infusion nurse also encounters patients who require subcutaneous (SC) and intraspinal infusions. SC infusion therapy is increasingly common, while intraspinal infusions are less common but clearly a high-risk type of infusion that demands clinician competency and organizational policies and procedures. Competency includes knowledge of anatomy and physiology, infusion administration, and management techniques aimed at maintaining access and reducing the risk of complications (Gorski et al., 2016, p. S118).

After reading this chapter, the reader will be able to:

- Identify indications for SC and intraspinal infusions
- Discuss SC and intraspinal access device care and management
- Identify potential complications

SC TISSUE ACCESS AND INFUSION

SC administration of medications or fluids is an increasingly common infusion route in home infusion therapy. A number of medications may be administered via the SC route including opioid infusions for pain management, immunoglobulin therapy, ondansetron, deferoxamine, and terbutaline. Although rarely administered as SC in current home infusion practice, SC administration of the antibiotics ceftriaxone and ertapenem appear to be bioequivalent to IV administration (Arthur, 2015; Jin et al., 2015). In a study of palliative care practice, the most commonly SC-administered medications were hydromorphone, haloperidol, and midazolam; however, the administration method studied was bolus SC delivery rather than infusion (Bartz et al., 2014). A systematic review was undertaken to analyze the advantages and disadvantages of SC, IV, and intramuscular administration in head-to-head comparative studies (Jin et al., 2015). The researchers suggest that when safety and efficacy of two injection routes are equivalent (e.g., IV and SC), clinicians should give more consideration to patient preference and pharmacoeconomics to promote optimal treatment adherence, improve patient experience or satisfaction, and reduce overall health care costs.

Advantages to the SC route include ease of access compared to cannulating a vein—most patients have adequate SC tissue with a variety of available locations—and minimal skill is required allowing some patients and caregivers to learn SC access (Arthur, 2015). Limitations and potential contraindications to the SC route may include poor circulation, limited SC tissue, and bleeding or coagulation disorders.

With IV administration, medications or fluids are injected directly into the bloodstream and there is no need for tissue absorption that is required with SC injection. Although there is a slower rate of achieving the maximum concentration of a medication, there is similar bioavailability by both the SC and the IV administration routes (Arthur, 2015). Human recombinant hyaluronidase (HRH) is a medication that can be used to facilitate and hasten the absorption of SC fluids or medications. The HRH is injected just before or with the SC agent. The current INS standards recommend consideration of hyaluronidase to facilitate the dispersion and absorption of hydration fluids and other SC-administered drugs (Gorski et al., 2016, p. S123).

Fast Facts in a Nutshell

The SC tissue is located beneath the dermal layer of the skin and contains blood vessels, nerves, and adipose tissue. Fat tissue in the SC tissue contains numerous blood vessels allowing for diffusion of the SC fluids into the circulation (Figure 6.1).

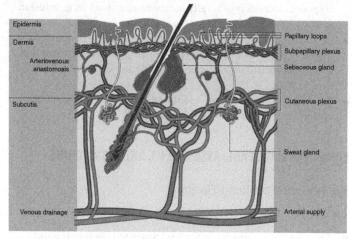

Figure 6.1 Anatomy of subcutaneous tissue. *Source: Young, O'Dowd, and Woodford (2014). Used with permission.*

PATIENT SELECTION CONSIDERATIONS

General guidelines for home SC infusion in relation to the patient include:

- The patient and family are motivated and willing and capable of participating in self-infusion management.
- The patient is clinically stable.
- The home environment is safe, clean, with adequate refrigeration space, and the patient has ready access to a telephone.
- Reimbursement is verified.

More specific guidelines for patients who may be candidates for SC infusion include:

- Patients with limited or difficult venous access and the prescribed medication or fluid is appropriate for SC administration.
- Patients with evidence of moderate dehydration: SC infusion is an alternative to IV administration of isotonic fluids. SC infusion of isotonic hydration fluids is called "hypodermoclysis."

Hypodermoclysis is generally indicated as a short-term infusion therapy, generally for 2 to 3 days or less (see Chapter 8).

■ Patients requiring pain management: SC infusion of opioid drugs (e.g., morphine and hydromorphone) for pain management is a common practice in palliative care and hospice settings (see Chapter 12).

■ Patients requiring immunoglobulin therapy: SC infusion is an option for some patients (see Chapter 14).

COMPREHENSIVE CARE, ASSESSMENT, AND MONITORING

Site Assessment and Device Placement

Site Selection

■ Any area where there is adequate SC tissue and the skin is intact (no evidence of bruising, irritation, or scarring) can be used.

■ Most common sites are abdomen (avoid area around navel because of blood vessel proximity), anterior thighs, subclavicular chest wall, upper back, and upper arm.

Site Preparation

■ Wash visibly dirty skin with soap and water.

■ Skin antisepsis: Antiseptic agents are the same as those used for IV preparation, including chlorhexidine–alcohol solutions, 70% alcohol, or povidone-iodine (Gorski et al., 2016).

Device/Type Placement

■ Review and follow the manufacturer's directions for use with any device.

■ Use small gauge (24–27 gauge) infusion device.

■ If using an over-the-needle catheter, enter the SC tissue at a 30- to 45-degree angle, depending on the thickness of the tissue.

■ Specially designed SC sets are inserted at a 90-degree angle.

■ Aspirate to ensure that there is no blood return, which confirms that the device is in the tissue and not in a small blood vessel (Gorski et al., 2016).

Dressing and Securement

■ A transparent semipermeable dressing is placed over the site, which allows for continuous site observation and assessment.

Infusion Guidelines

Administration Rates and Methods

- Hypodermoclysis: Use of a manual flow regulator is recommended (see Chapter 7); an infusion rate of 1,500 mL over 24 hours, which is approximately 60 mL per hour. More than one site may be simultaneously used for larger volumes.
- Medication administration: Use an electronic infusion device. Although the optimal upper limit of an SC infusion rate is unknown, an infusion rate of 3 to 5 mL per hour is common (Gorski et al., 2016).
- SC immunoglobulin administration: Syringe pumps are often used; in some cases, patients are taught to manually push the infusion (Gorski et al., 2016, p. S123).

Site Rotation

- Hypodermoclysis: Change the site after 1.5 to 2 L of fluid have been administered in a single site. Depending on tolerance and site assessment, the site may need to be rotated earlier.
- Medication administration: Every 7 days and as clinically indicated, based on the integrity of the access site.
- SC immunoglobulin administration: Limit infusion volume to no more than 30 mL per site (see Chapter 14).
- Assessment of individual patient tolerance is an important aspect when considering frequency of site rotation.

Monitoring for Complications

Complications related to SC infusions are generally minor. Some edema is expected with hypodermoclysis but will subside as the fluid is absorbed. The infusion rate may need to be reduced. The use of a plastic-type device instead of a steel needle should be considered. Monitor the SC access site with each home visit:

- Observe site for erythema, swelling, leaking of fluid, bleeding, bruising, or patient complaints of burning or itching at the site (Gorski et al., 2016).
- The most common problem is local inflammation/pain/discomfort at the needle site; may be caused by highly concentrated drug solutions or too rapid infusion rate. Intervene by increasing the frequency of site rotation, changing concentration or infusion

rates. Treat inflammation with cool compresses, and avoid harsh soaps or lotions in the area.
- HRH reactions: Redness, pain, anaphylactic-like or allergic reactions.

PATIENT EDUCATION: KEY POINTS

- SC access device
- Plan of care for infusion therapy
- Check site at least twice per day
- Report any redness, swelling, or pain to the nurse
- SC access device placement, site rotation procedure, and infusion management if self-administration is the goal of care

INTRASPINAL CATHETERS

Intraspinal catheters commonly refer to the epidural or intrathecal catheter. In the home setting, patients who require intraspinal catheter and infusions are usually those who have chronic pain of a malignant or nonmalignant nature. Opioid drugs and anesthetic agents are typically infused via the intraspinal catheter. Medications infused must be preservative free as preservatives are associated with neurotoxicity. Examples of medications that may be infused via an intraspinal catheter include preservative-free morphine, fentanyl, hydromorphone, ziconotide, clonidine, bupivacaine, and baclofen (Gorski et al., 2016).

Fast Facts in a Nutshell

Intraspinal access device care and infusion is not common in home care. Organizations must have policies and procedures in place before accepting patients requiring such infusions. Home care nurses must take responsibility and acquire the appropriate knowledge and skill before performing such procedures (American Nurses Association, 2014).

Spinal Anatomy

The spinal cord begins at the base of the skull, passes through the vertebral canal of the spinal column, and terminates at the first or second lumbar vertebra. The spinal cord is protected by the vertebrae and its ligaments and is surrounded by three protective membranes that also surround the brain (Drake, Vogl, & Mitchell, 2010):

- Pia mater: A delicate, cellular, and vascular membrane that adheres and tightly clings to the entire spinal cord
- Arachnoid mater: A nonvascular, spider web–like membrane that surrounds and is connected to the pia mater with filaments of connective tissue
- Dura mater: The fatty, tougher outermost membrane of the spinal cord

The space between the pia and the arachnoid mater is the intrathecal (or subarachnoid) space that contains the cerebrospinal fluid (CSF) that bathes and protects the spinal cord. The space outside of the dura mater and before the vertebral canal is called the "epidural space." The epidural space is a potential space with fatty tissue, vascular networks, and connective tissues; it becomes a true space when fluid is administered. The epidural space contains protruding nerve roots with dural sheaths (Figure 6.2). Due to the vascular network within the space, the epidural space is considered leukocytic, which reduces the risk of infection.

- Epidural drug infusion: When a drug is administered through a catheter placed in the epidural space, the drug must diffuse through the dura mater. Narcotics infused in this manner produce pain relief due to a direct effect on opiate receptors located in the dorsal horn. Because drug distribution is limited, there are fewer motor and sensory side effects with epidural infusion. Lower doses of analgesics are required than when systemically administered (e.g., IV, SC, or oral).
- Intrathecal infusion: Intrathecal administration puts the drug directly into the CSF where it bathes the dorsal horn of the spinal cord and is available to bind with opioid receptors. Drugs administered into the intrathecal space are given in much smaller doses—about 1/10th of the epidural dose.
- Once drug is in the CSF, drug flows in two directions: Actively and primarily to the brain ("rostral" flow—this is the direction of CSF flow) and passively and minimally toward the base of the spine (Stearns & Brant, 2010).

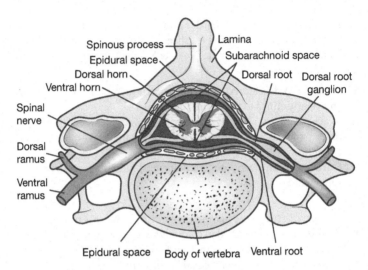

Figure 6.2 Vertebral canal.

Types of Catheters

- Temporary—A percutaneously placed catheter used for a trial period, usually less than 2 weeks due to increased risk for infection and catheter dislodgement or migration (Stearns & Brant, 2010); may be an epidural or an intrathecal catheter. During the trial, the patient's clinical response to epidural drug infusion is assessed. If the trial is successful, the plan would include placement of a long-term catheter.

- Long-term catheters include the subcutaneously tunneled catheter that exits usually in the abdominal area or an implanted epidural port that is accessed using a noncoring needle. These types of catheters are used most often for long-term epidural infusions.

- Long-term totally implanted catheter and programmable infusion pump are used for epidural or intrathecal infusion. The drug is injected directly into the pump using a noncoring needle. The pump can be programmed externally using a sensor wand.

Fast Facts in a Nutshell

Make sure that home care referral information includes specific type of catheter placement; some clinicians may inadvertently confuse epidural and intrathecal terminology. Best practice is to obtain and include copy of the operative procedure in the home care patient record.

PATIENT SELECTION CONSIDERATIONS

General guidelines for home intraspinal infusions in relation to the patient include:

- The patient and family are motivated and willing and capable of participating in self-infusion management.
- The patient is clinically stable.
- The home environment is safe, clean, with adequate refrigeration space, and the patient has ready access to a telephone.
- Reimbursement is verified.

Specific clinical indications for intraspinal infusion include:

- Absence of contraindications to epidural or catheter placement (coagulopathies, sepsis, and CNS structural pathology)
- Chronic pain of malignant or nonmalignant origin

COMPREHENSIVE CARE, ASSESSMENT, AND MONITORING

Site Assessment and Site Care

- Assess for signs of insertion site infection or epidural abscess: back pain, site tenderness, erythema, swelling, drainage, fever, malaise, neck stiffness, progressive numbness.
- Assess dressing for intactness and absence of moisture/leakage.
- Assess for catheter migration by measuring external catheter length.
- Site care:
  - Short-term catheters: Routine dressing changes are not recommended due to the risk of dislodgement;

chlorhexidine-impregnated dressings are often used to reduce risk for infection.

■ Tunneled and accessed implanted port sites: Site care and dressing changes per organizational policies; usually every 5 to 7 days when a transparent semipermeable membrane dressing is used.

■ Use strict aseptic technique.

■ Povidone-iodine is used for site care antiseptic agent; alcohol is never used for site preparation, cleansing the catheter hub, or during dressing changes due to its potential deleterious effect as a neurotoxin.

■ Ensure that catheter is secured to skin to avoid accidental dislodgement.

Fast Facts in a Nutshell

Any accidental intraspinal system "disconnects" should be immediately reported to the anesthesiologist. A break in the system allows the risk for intraluminal migration of microbes and increases the risk for infection.

Infusion Guidelines

■ Minimize the number of times that the intraspinal infusion system is entered; for example, limit the frequency of drug reservoir changes.

■ Use strict aseptic technique, with mask and sterile gloves.

■ Use only preservative-free solutions and medications as preservatives may be neurotoxic.

■ Verify that the catheter is an intraspinal catheter by tracing the catheter from the cap to the exit site; label tubing/catheter.

■ Filter use: Use a 0.2 μm surfactant-free filter for intraspinal drug infusion. Change in accordance with manufacturer's recommendations.

■ Aspirate catheter prior to initiating infusion (Gorski et al., 2016):

   ■ Epidural catheters: Minimal fluid return is indicative of placement in the epidural space; if more than 0.5 mL obtained, do not inject medication and notify physician.

- Intrathecal catheters: Free-flowing clear fluid is indicative of placement in the intrathecal space; blood in the aspirate is indicative of migration into a blood vessel and if present, do not inject medication and notify physician.
- Intraspinal catheters are not routinely flushed.

Monitoring for Complications

Note: This section focuses specifically on intraspinal catheter–related complications. Complications related to intraspinal analgesic infusion, including urinary retention, respiratory depression, and pruritus are covered in Chapter 12.

Infection

- Local site signs/symptoms (s/s) include redness, swelling, drainage, warmth, or soreness at exit site of catheter.
- Epidural or intrathecal space infection: s/s include diffuse back pain/tenderness, pain during bolus injection, inadequate pain relief, sensory or motor changes, and/or fever.
- Acute bacterial infection: fever, headache, nuchal rigidity, altered mental status, convulsions.
- *Immediately* report any s/s of infection.

Catheter Migration/Dislodgment

- Catheter migration, especially with the use of temporary catheters, can occur at any time and is a common occurrence.
- Intrathecal migrates into epidural space—signs include inadequate pain relief, no reduction in pain with increased doses, and no CSF aspirate (intrathecal).
- Epidural migrates into intrathecal—look for increased drug side effects and aspiration of CSF.
- Intravascular migration—inadequate pain relief, unexplained increased in opioid side effects, s/s of local anesthetic toxicity, and aspiration of free-flowing blood.
- Reduce risk of catheter migration by following care and maintenance guidelines listed previously.
- *Immediately* report any evidence of catheter migration or dislodgement.

PATIENT EDUCATION: KEY POINTS

- Intraspinal catheter: rationale, placement, expected effects
- Plan of care for infusion therapy
- Check site at least twice per day
- Report any redness, swelling, signs of leakage, or site tenderness/pain to the nurse immediately
- Report any changes in condition such as change in pain level, increased drowsiness, and weakness to the nurse immediately
- Safe handling of infusion pump to reduce risk of pulling/catheter dislodgement
- Patients with implanted infusion pump system: Caution with active repetitive bending or twisting of spine as these movements may increase the risk for catheter damage or dislodgement; increased pain and withdrawal symptoms may indicate problems (Prager et al., 2014)

TEST YOUR KNOWLEDGE

1. Hyaluronidase may be used with SC infusions to:
   a. Decrease the risk of SC side effects
   b. Facilitate drug absorption
   c. Decrease the dosage of SC drug infusion
   d. Increase the rate of SC infusion
2. SC tissue is located below:
   a. The dermis
   b. The skin
   c. The epidermis
   d. Fatty tissue
3. The infusion rate for hypodermoclysis is limited to:
   a. 60 mL per hour
   b. 75 mL per hour
   c. 100 mL per hour
   d. 125 mL per hour
4. The space between the pia and the arachnoid mater:
   a. Is a potential space
   b. Is called the dura mater
   c. Is called the epidural space
   d. Contains CSF
5. When are site care and dressing changes on a temporary epidural catheter generally done?

   a. Every 2 days
   b. Every 5 to 7 days
   c. As needed
   d. Site care and dressing changes are not routinely done
6. Signs that may be indicative of an intrathecal catheter migrating into the epidural space include:
   a. Inadequate pain relief
   b. Increased opioid side effects
   c. Fever
   d. Nuccal rigidity

ANSWERS

1. b
2. a
3. a
4. d
5. d
6. a

References

American Nurses Association. (2014). *Home health nursing: Scope and standards of practice* (2nd ed.). Silver Spring, MD: Author.

Arthur, A. O. (2015). Innovations in subcutaneous infusions. *Journal of Infusion Nursing, 38*(3), 179–187.

Bartz, L., Klein, C., Seifert, A., Herget, I. Ostgathe, C., & Stiel, S. (2014). Subcutaneous administration of drugs in palliative care: Results of a systematic observational study. *Journal of Pain and Symptom Management, 48*(4), 540–547.

Drake, R. L., Vogl, W., & Mitchell, A. W. (2010). *Gray's anatomy for students* (2nd ed.). St. Louis, MO: Elsevier.

Gorski, L. A., Hadaway, L., Hagle, M., McGoldrick, M., Orr, M., & Doellman, D. (2016). Infusion therapy standards of practice. *Journal of Infusion Nursing, 39*(1S), S1–S159.

Jin, J. F., Zhu, L. L., Chen, M., Xu, H. M., Wang, H. F., Feng, X. Q., . . . Zhou, Q. (2015). The optimal choice of medication administration route regarding intravenous, intramuscular, and subcutaneous injection. *Patient Preference and Adherence, 9*, 923–942.

Prager, J., Deer, T., Levy, R. Bruel, B., Buchser, E., Caraway, D., . . . Stearns, L. (2014). Best practices for intrathecal drug delivery. *Neuromodulation, 17*(4), 354–372.

Stearns, C. K., & Brant, J. M. (2010). Intraspinal access and medication administration. In M. Alexander, A. Corrigan, L. A. Gorski, J. Hankins, &

R. Perucca (Eds.), *Infusion nursing: An evidence-based approach* (3rd ed., pp. 535–539). St. Louis, MO: Saunders/Elsevier.

Young, B., O'Dowd, G., & Woodford, P. (2014). *Wheater's functional histology: A text and colour atlas* (6th ed.). Edinburgh, Scotland: Churchill Livingstone/Elsevier.

III

Principles of Delivering Infusion Therapy Within the Home Environment

7

Infusion Administration Methods and Issues

The infusion administration method is selected and based upon multiple factors including the type of infusion, the frequency of administration, infusion rate requirements, drug stability in solution, patient safety and lifestyle concerns, patient preference, and reimbursement. Patient safety is maximized by teaching the patient and family how to administer the infusion therapy, how to use an infusion pump, how to identify potential problems, and when/whom to call with problems. For patients who require a continuous infusion and are "hooked up" to an infusion pump 24 hours a day, teaching must also address how to manage activities of daily living. Other issues related to infusion administration addressed in this chapter include the administration set and filtration.

After reading this chapter, the reader will be able to:

- Identify advantages and disadvantages for common infusion administration methods
- Identify appropriate use of infusion pumps
- Discuss issues that impact patient selection for any given infusion administration method
- Identify key points for patient education

NONINFUSION PUMP METHODS: IV PUSH AND GRAVITY DRIP

IV Push

Direct injection of an intravenous (IV) medication, called "IV push," is the administration of the medication in a syringe directly into the patient's vascular access device (VAD) or through the injection port of a continuous infusion. In home care, IV push is used most often for certain antimicrobials, including some in the cephalosporin group (e.g., ceftriaxone, cefazolin, and cefapime). Other examples of medications that may be administered by IV push include antiemetics (e.g., ondansetron) or diuretics (e.g., furosemide).

Advantages to IV push administration include less administration time, cost-effectiveness in terms of supplies, and a relatively simple administration method. However, nurses often administer IV push medications too rapidly (Carter, Gelchion, Saitta, & Clark, 2011; Institute for Safe Medication Practices, 2015). It is important to recognize the risk of "speed shock," a systemic reaction that occurs when a medication is too rapidly administered into the circulation. Symptoms include dizziness, facial flushing, headache, and medication-specific symptoms that can progress to chest tightness, hypotension, irregular pulse, and anaphylaxis (Phillips & Gorski, 2014). It is critically important to administer IV push medications over the appropriate time frame. The medication syringe should be labeled with the administration time (e.g., "administer over 3 to 5 minutes").

Fast Facts in a Nutshell

Nurses who administer IV push medications without use of a watch or second hand tend to underestimate the time that has passed and will often administer at a rate faster than recommended. Always use a watch or clock with a second hand or with a digital display of minutes and seconds; use of the timer function on a cell phone is another suggestion. This is also a critical aspect of patient education for patients or caregivers who self-administer (Figure 7.1).

Gravity Drip

Gravity infusion is a common method used to deliver intermittent medications. It is cost-effective, using an infusion container (e.g., minibag with antibiotic) and simple IV tubing. An IV pole is required or,

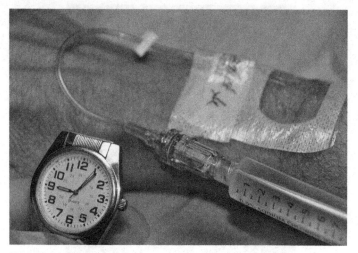

Figure 7.1 Administering an IV push medication. *Source: Photograph courtesy of Sherry Lokken, RN.*

Note: To reduce the risk of complications associated with rapid administration, always use a watch or other timer device to ensure an appropriate administration rate.

IV, intravenous.

alternatively, the infusion container can be hung from a home structure such as a drapery rod. For some antibiotics, the medication is contained in a separate compartment with a premeasured drug and diluent that is mixed just prior to administration (Figure 7.2). This method is used for medications that have a limited shelf-life after admixture.

The IV drop rate must be calculated. Necessary information for calculation includes the volume of the infusion, the time frame for infusion in minutes, and the number of drops per milliliter as listed on the container of the IV tubing set. Calculate the IV drop rate as follows:

---

volume (mL)/ time (min) × drop factor (drops/mL) = drop rate

Example:

50 mL of fluid is administered over 30 minutes;
the drop factor of the IV tubing is 10 drops/mL

(50 mL/30 min) × (10 drops/mL) = 16.6 or
17 drops per minute

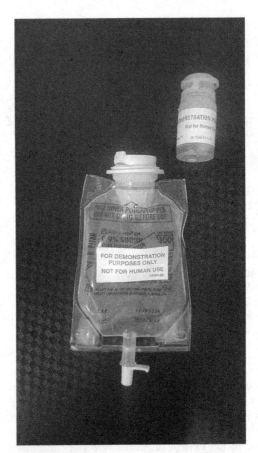

Figure 7.2 Use-activated container.

Note: In accordance with the specific manufacturer's directions for use, the medication container is connected to the port of the solution bag and the medication is mixed with the diluent. It is used for infusions that have a limited shelf-life once admixed (e.g., ertapenem).

A manual flow regulator is often used in lieu of the built-in roller clamp of the IV tubing. The regulator allows the nurse or patient to set the flow rate in milliliters per hour (Figure 7.3). Advantages may include easier regulation, more consistent flow, less drifting of flow compared to using the roller clamp, and less risk of accidental free-flow. However, the accuracy is about the same as the roller clamp (± 10%).

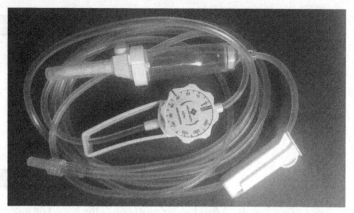

Figure 7.3 Administration set with manual flow regulator.

Note: It may be used in lieu of the built-in roller clamp of the IV tubing, allowing the nurse or patient to set the flow rate in milliliters per hour.

For patients who require multiple doses per day, the IV tubing is changed every 24 hours as recommended by the Infusion Nurses Society (INS; Gorski et al., 2016). From a procedural standpoint, the infusion is stopped when the infusion container is empty but fluid still remains in the drip chamber. With subsequent infusions within the 24-hour period, a new infusion container is aseptically respiked to the existing tubing.

Patient Selection Considerations: IV Push and Gravity Drip

- Safety is a concern due to rate management and risk for reactions with IV push.
- Gravity drip is a more complex procedure as it involves more steps in accordance with attention to infection prevention including maintenance of aseptic technique. Key steps include:
  - Removing the protective cap from the tubing spike
  - Inserting the tubing spike into the infusion container
  - Filling the drip chamber and priming the IV tubing while protecting the male luer end of the tubing from touch contamination
  - Managing the infusion rate by drop counting

Fast Facts in a Nutshell

A manual flow regulator is not an equivalent to an infusion pump. The drops should be counted to match the set rate on the dial. Such devices enhance the ease of infusion but do not take away the need to monitor the flow rate whether by the home care nurse or the patient/caregiver.

Fast Facts in a Nutshell

It is critically important that the male luer end of the tubing be protected with a new, sterile cover that is aseptically attached (Gorski et al., 2016). If there is any contamination of the male luer end of the tubing, it should be discarded as it is a source for contamination and it increases the risk for a bloodstream infection.

INFUSION PUMP ADMINISTRATION: ELASTOMERIC BALLOON "PUMPS"

The elastomeric balloon pump is a portable device that consists of an elastomeric reservoir, or balloon (Figure 7.4). Made of a soft rubberized material that is inflated to a predetermined volume, the balloon is encapsulated inside a rigid, transparent container. The balloon exerts positive pressure to administer the medication; control over fluid flow rate is maintained by IV tubing with varying tubing diameters. These devices are used to deliver a variety of infusion therapies, including IV antibiotics, chemotherapy, and analgesics. Volumes range from 50 to 250 mL. Elastomeric pumps can infuse at rates from 0.5 to 500 mL/hr.

Patient Selection Considerations: Elastomeric Balloon Pumps

- A portable, disposable, nongravity-dependent infusion device that is often ideal for active patients or children who continue to work or go to school
- Easier to learn compared to gravity infusion as the steps of bag spiking and rate monitoring are eliminated

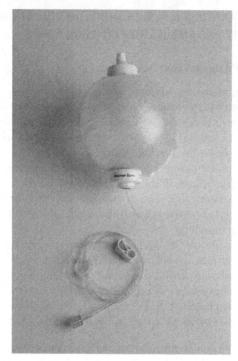

Figure 7.4 Elastomeric pump. *Source: Photo courtesy of Halyard Health, Alpharetta, Georgia.*

Note: These pumps come in a variety of volumes and may be used to administer medications such as antibiotics, chemotherapy, and analgesics.

Fast Facts in a Nutshell

Flow rate at the beginning of the infusion is faster than the rate at the end of the infusion due to variations in pressure within the stretched elastomeric membrane (Skryabina & Dunn, 2006). For patients who are sensitive to the infusion rate, this may be a concern. For example, "red man syndrome" is an adverse reaction of vancomycin associated with the infusion rate (see Chapter 9). Temperature affects performance; when the infusate is cold, the flow rate is slower. Instruct patients to remove the filled device from the refrigerator several hours before the infusion, based on manufacturer's directions for use and pharmacy instructions.

ELECTRONIC INFUSION PUMP ADMINISTRATION: SYRINGE, STATIONARY, AND AMBULATORY INFUSION PUMPS

Syringe and Stationary Electronic Pumps

Syringe pumps use a traditional syringe as the solution container, which is filled with prescribed medication and positioned in a special pump designed to hold it. Syringe pumps control the infusion rate by drive speed and syringe size, thus eliminating the variables of the drop rate. In home care, syringe pumps are used for delivery of antibiotics, subcutaneous immune globulin infusions, and small-volume IV therapy. The volume of the syringe pump is limited to the size of the syringe; a 60-mL syringe is often used. However, the syringe can be as small as 5 mL. The tubing usually is a single, uninterrupted length of kink-resistant tubing.

Stationary electronic pumps are mounted on an IV pole. They allow for large infusion volumes and a wide range of infusion rates. They may be less expensive than other pumps. Mobility is an issue and these pumps are usually used for longer, larger intermittent infusions (e.g., amphotericin B, IV immunoglobulin [IVIG] infusions, and continuous infusions in a patient with limited mobility).

Patient Selection Considerations: Syringe and Stationary Electronic Infusion Pumps

- Must be able to learn the steps of loading the syringe and using the pump correctly
- Nurse-administered infusions when patient independence is not appropriate due to infusate risks (e.g., IVIG infusion)

Ambulatory Electronic Infusion Devices (EIDs)

Ambulatory EIDs are lightweight and compact infusion pumps that are capable of delivering most infusion therapies including continuous infusions (e.g., chemotherapy and inotropes), intermittent antibiotic therapy, analgesic infusions with patient-controlled analgesia (PCA), and continuous infusions with tapering functions (e.g., parenteral nutrition [PN]). For intermittent antimicrobial infusions, a "keep vein open rate" is programmed to maintain flow between the drug administrations. Features include programmable memory, lock-out functions for safety, and alarms. "Smart pumps" that include drug libraries are available. Ambulatory pumps function on a battery system that requires recharging or replacement of disposable batteries. The pump along with the infusion container is placed in a pouch or backpack, providing the patient with full mobility during the infusion.

Patient Selection Considerations: Ambulatory EIDs

- Patients who require frequent (every 4- to 6-hour) dosing or continuous infusions
- Those who lack manual dexterity, who have impaired cognitive function, and/or are unwilling or unable to learn the necessary techniques for self-administration, and those who lack a support person at home

Fast Facts in a Nutshell

Although the infusion pharmacy usually makes initial decisions regarding the best infusion method or device for the type of infusion therapy, the home care nurse may also make recommendations. After assessing the patient and home situation, the nurse may advocate for a better method; for example, recommending an elastomeric pump to facilitate the patient's independence, mobility, and return to work. Collaboration between the home care nurse and home infusion pharmacist is an important aspect of home infusion therapy, contributing to positive patient outcomes as well as health care provider satisfaction.

Decision Making: The Best Infusion Method

The initial decision regarding the best infusion method or device for the type of infusion therapy is generally made by the home infusion pharmacy. A number of factors that drive infusion administration method choice include:

- Drug or infusion solution:
  - Compatibility with infusion device (e.g., elastomeric)
  - Need for accurate rate control (e.g., continuous infusion requiring an EID)
  - Safety of rapid infusion (e.g., IV push)
- Drug stability in solution:
  - May limit ability to use an ambulatory, programmable pump because the infusion container is generally prepared for a

24-hour infusion; for example, intermittent doses of ampicillin have limited stability of only 4 to 8 hours once admixed (Gahart, Nazareno, & Ortega, 2016)

- Patient safety and lifestyle concerns and patient preference
- Cost/reimbursement:
  - Some insurance companies will have restrictions (e.g., some will not cover an elastomeric device)

Fast Facts in a Nutshell

Safe use and operation of infusion pumps, for example, may be affected by temperature extremes, presence of children and pets, dirt and dust, poor lighting, and limited space (Hilbers, de Vries, & Geertsma, 2013). As home-based care continues to grow, it is recommended and expected that manufacturers who develop medical equipment for use in the home attend to such risks during the design process.

OTHER INFUSION ADMINISTRATION ISSUES: ADMINISTRATION SETS AND FILTRATION

The INS standards (Gorski et al., 2016, pp. S84–S85) provide guidance on filtration and how often to change the administration set, commonly called "tubing," as follows:

- Intermittent infusions: Change the set every 24 hours. Make sure the male luer end of the tubing is not touched and that a sterile, compatible cap is placed on the end when used for more than one infusion per day. When systems such as elastomeric pumps are used, the tubing is inherent to the container with the whole unit discarded after use.
- Parenteral nutrition: Change the set every 24 hours. If IV fat emulsions are administered as a separate infusion, change that tubing every 12 hours.
- Continuous infusions: Change the administration set no more often than every 96 hours. With home infusion, the infusion container may provide a week's worth of medication (e.g., morphine infusion); while not addressed in the INS standards,

it is not atypical to change the entire infusion system (drug reservoir and tubing) on a weekly basis.

- Filtration:
  - The purpose of filtration is to prevent the administration of particulate matter, air, microorganisms, or endotoxins that may be in the infusion system. Filters are available as separate add-on devices or as in-line components as part of the IV administration set. The filter is changed with the administration set.
  - PN and separate lipid infusions are always filtered. A 1.2-μm filter is required for PN solutions with lipids or lipid infusions alone. A 0.2-μm filter is used for PN solutions without lipids.
  - Intraspinal infusions are filtered using a surfactant-free 0.2-μm filter.
  - Some medications require filtration based upon manufacturer's guidelines (e.g., infliximab and some immunoglobulin infusions). Always refer to the drug package insert and consult with the infusion pharmacist regarding any filtration questions.

PATIENT EDUCATION: KEY POINTS

General Guidelines

Ensure that copy of the infusion pump manual is in the home:
- May also provide additional personalized teaching handouts
- Consider use of online infusion pump patient education, if available

Instruct in:
- Whom to call with problems, alarms, or questions (home care nurse vs. home infusion pharmacy)
- Infusion pump profile (e.g., drug infused, rate or duration of each dose and when each dose kicks in for intermittent antibiotics, duration of infusion, and any tapering time for total PN)—leave written copy in home
- Alarms and actions to take:
  - How to change the battery, if used
  - Check the pump and IV reservoir/cassette one to two times per day
    - Check that numbers on the pump screen are increasing (or decreasing) as the infusion progresses
    - Check that the volume of fluid in the drug reservoir is decreasing

- Activities of daily living issues, especially for patients on continuous infusions
- Bathing or showering, if allowed. Teach patient how to secure and protect infusion pump and IV catheter/dressing from moisture
- How to dress and undress, handling IV tubing and threading through clothing, and avoiding tension (and potential dislodgement) at IV site
- Importance of picking up and carrying the pump when ambulating

Infusion Pump Risk Reduction Strategies for Patients Using Infusion Pumps at Home

The Food and Drug Administration (FDA) has provided guidance to both clinicians and patients related to safe infusion pump use. Nurses and physicians can refer patients to the FDA website (www.fda.gov/ MedicalDevices/ProductsandMedicalProcedures/GeneralHospital DevicesandSupplies/InfusionPumps/ucm205412.htm) or print out this information to guide patient education:

Reduce risk: plan ahead

- Work with your home health nurse (or other outpatient antimicrobial therapy [OPAT] team member) to develop a back-up plan in case of an infusion pump failure.
- Know if your plan includes calling 911.
- Know where your infusion pump back-up battery is located and how to access an emergency power supply, if applicable.
- Refer to Home Healthcare Medical Devices: Infusion Therapy— Getting the Most out of Your Pump (www.fda.gov/Medical Devices/ProductsandMedicalProcedures/HomeHealthand Consumer/ucm070208.htm) for more information.

Learn about your infusion pump and medication. Ask your home health care provider:

- About the infusion pump:
  - What is the name of my infusion pump?
  - Is this infusion pump already set up?
  - Do I need to look at anything on the infusion pump to make sure it is correct? If so, what?
  - How do I start and stop the infusion pump?

- Do I need training to use this infusion pump?
  - Will any electrical items in my home interfere with my pump?
- About your medication:
  - What is the name of my medication?
  - What does the medication do? How should it make me feel?
  - What are the side effects?
  - What is the dose of my medication?
  - How long should my medication take to complete?
  - Can there be medication left in my tubing or in my bag when the infusion pump stops?
- What to do when there are problems:
  - What should I look for if I am getting too much medication too fast?
  - What should I look for if I am getting too little medication?
  - Whom should I call with questions or problems?
  - What should I do if the power goes out?

Check:
- Make sure you can read the infusion pump's displays and hear the alarms, if applicable.
- Verify the settings when starting or changing the rate of a medication or fluid, if applicable.
- If they are not correct, or if you have questions, call your home health provider.

Report problems—call your home health care provider to obtain further instructions if:
- The infusion pump appears broken or damaged or has small chips or cracks
- An unfamiliar alarm sounds or is displayed
- An alarm is unable to be cleared to which you have been trained to respond

You are also encouraged to file a voluntary report (www.fda.gov/MedicalDevices/ProductsandMedicalProcedures/GeneralHospitalDevicesandSupplies/InfusionPumps/ucm202503.htm) with the FDA for any problems you may encounter with the infusion pump.

TEST YOUR KNOWLEDGE

1. The simplest and most cost-effective infusion administration method for a patient who requires a daily infusion of ceftriaxone is:
   a. IV push
   b. Elastomeric pump
   c. Gravity drip
   d. Stationary bedside infusion pump

2. Symptoms of "speed shock" associated with too rapid IV administration include:
   a. Headache and nausea
   b. Dizziness and facial flushing
   c. Nausea and vomiting
   d. Nausea and diarrhea

3. Calculate the drop rate per minute for a patient who requires an infusion that includes 100 mL of ceftriaxone over 30 minutes. The drop factor of the administration set is 15 drops/mL.
   a. 50 drops per minute
   b. 75 drops per minute
   c. 100 drops per minute
   d. 200 drops per minute

4. Elastomeric infusion devices may be used for administration of:
   a. Parenteral nutrition
   b. Dobutamine infusions
   c. Chemotherapy infusions
   d. Immunoglobulin infusions

5. The use of an ambulatory infusion pump is definitely limited by:
   a. Patient preference
   b. Physician preference
   c. Drug stability in solution
   d. Cost

6. Filtration is required for:
   a. Most chemotherapy drugs
   b. Parenteral nutrition
   c. Most antibiotics
   d. Morphine infusions

ANSWERS

1. a
2. b
3. a
4. c
5. c
6. b

References

Carter, A., Gelchion, K., Saitta, P., & Clark, D. (2011). Dyeing to identify IV medication errors: A clinical nurse specialist group identifies factors contributing to IV push medication errors, and the resulting housewide education initiative. *Clinical Nurse Specialist*, *25*(3), 140–152.

Gahart, B. L., Nazareno, A. R., & Ortega, M. Q. (2016). *Gahart's 2016 intravenous medications: A handbook for nurses and health professionals* (32nd ed.). St. Louis, MO: Elsevier.

Gorski, L. A., Hadaway, L., Hagle, M., McGoldrick, M., Orr, M., & Doellman, D. (2016). Infusion therapy standards of practice. *Journal of Infusion Nursing*, *39*(1S), S1–S159.

Hilbers, E. S. M., de Vries, C. G. J. C. A., & Geertsma, R. E. (2013). Medical technology at home: Safety-related items in technical documentation. *International Journal of Technology Assessment in Health Care*, *29*(1), 20–26.

Institute for Safe Medication Practices. (2015). ISMP safe practice guidelines for adult IV push medications. Retrieved from http://www.ismp.org/Tools/guidelines/ivsummitpush/ivpushmedguidelines.pdf

Phillips, L., & Gorski, L. A. (2014). *Manual of IV therapeutics: Evidence-based practice for infusion therapy*. Philadelphia, PA: F.A. Davis.

Skryabina, E. A., & Dunn, T. S. (2006). Disposable infusion pumps. *American Journal of Health System Pharmacists*, *63*(13), 1260–1268.

8

Fluid Administration: Managing Dehydration

A mong the older adult population, a significant risk is that of dehydration affecting 20% to 30% of older adults (Miller, 2015). The consequences and complications of dehydration are prevented when early signs are identified and promptly treated. Untreated dehydration will progress to inability to control temperature, inability to sweat, development of fever, and diminished cardiac output (Miller, 2015). Although most patients with early signs of dehydration can be managed with increasing oral intake, those with moderate dehydration may benefit from infusion therapy. Besides the older and chronically ill population, other patient populations that may require infusion fluid replacement to prevent dehydration include pregnant women with hyperemesis gravidarum and patients who are undergoing chemotherapy. Home treatment has been found successful in reducing the risk for rehospitalization and emergency room visits (Konrad et al., 2016).

After reading this chapter, the reader will be able to:

- Discuss the risks and presentation of dehydration
- Summarize patient selection criteria for home infusion of fluids
- Describe key aspects of subcutaneous (SC) and intravenous (IV) fluid administration
- Summarize components of comprehensive care, assessment, and monitoring

DEHYDRATION: AN OVERVIEW

Dehydration is defined by a decline in total body water. The most common type of dehydration is isotonic dehydration resulting from an equal loss of water and electrolytes (Miller, 2015). Causes include diarrhea, vomiting, or inadequate fluid intake. Hypertonic dehydration is a result of excessive sodium in the extracellular fluid, a result of diuretics or inadequate fluid intake. Older adults are at higher risk for dehydration due to a number of factors that include natural changes associated with aging. These include a decreased percentage of total body water (60% in younger adults to 40% in older adults), decreased muscle mass (muscles store a large amount of water), decreased capacity to concentrate urine, and a decrease in the sensation of thirst. Other risk factors include age greater than 85 years, dependence on others for feeding and eating, dementia, presence of an infection, four or more chronic conditions, four or more medications, taking diuretics, vomiting/diarrhea, and prior episodes of dehydration (Mentes, 2012). A medication review is very important as polypharmacy is often a significant contributing factor to dehydration (Miller, 2015).

Signs and symptoms of dehydration are often unreliable in older adults. A rapid weight loss over 1 to 2 weeks should signal the possibility of dehydration (Morley, 2015). Mild dehydration is categorized by a water loss equivalent to 1% of body weight and by symptoms that include headache, fatigue, weakness, dizziness, and lethargy. Moderate dehydration may include additional symptoms of dry mouth, decreased urine output, and decreased skin elasticity. Skin turgor in older adults is usually not reliable, but if done should be checked on the forehead.

In terms of laboratory studies, they are not always reliable indicators in older adults. For example, the blood urea nitrogen (BUN) to serum creatinine level (>20) is a common measure of dehydration but is not reliable in older adults because a multitude of other factors may cause an elevation such as aging muscle loss, presence of renal/heart failure, glucocorticoids, and increased protein intake (Morley, 2015). While the serum osmolality has been reported as the gold standard to diagnose dehydration (Miller, 2015), making the diagnosis of dehydration is actually quite challenging. A level of more than 295 mOsm/kg may indicate a hyperosmolar state and dehydration. Urinalysis may also be helpful providing information about specific gravity (high), color, and presence of leukocytes, nitrites, and blood, which may indicate a urinary tract infection that could be a cause of decreased fluid intake. In a Cochrane review, no tests were found to be consistently useful in diagnosing water-loss dehydration in older adults; the researchers assert that the following tests should *not* be used to diagnose dehydration: dry mouth, feeling thirsty, heart rate, and urine color and volume (Hooper et al., 2015). In a clinical article, the authors suggest clinical observations should be based on the patient history, physical assessment, laboratory values, and clinician experience (Armstrong, Kavouras, Walsh, & Roberts, 2016). Clearly, comprehensive assessment by the home care nurse in interprofessional collaboration with the physician and the pharmacist is essential in making the best decision in identification of and treatment of dehydration.

For patients with evidence suggesting severe dehydration such as fever, confusion, and little to no urination, hospitalization is recommended as it is considered a medical emergency (Miller, 2015). For patients with moderate dehydration, infusion fluid administration may be appropriate and hypodermoclysis is suggested.

Infusion Fluid Replacement: IV versus SC Administration

For younger adults with good vascular access or the presence of an existing vascular access device (VAD), the IV route is a more common infusion route. Patients with cancer who are experiencing side effects impacting fluid intake may have an implanted port or other central VAD (CVAD) that may be used for fluid replacement. Patients with conditions such as hyperemesis gravidarum may require longer courses of fluid replacement until symptoms recede and a peripheral or midline catheter (shorter term needs) or CVAD such as a peripherally inserted central catheter (PICC) is often placed for fluid needs.

Primarily used in the older adult with dehydration, SC infusion is an alternative to IV administration of isotonic fluids as presented in Chapter 6. SC infusion of hydration fluids is called "hypodermoclysis." Hypodermoclysis is generally indicated as a short-term infusion therapy, generally for 2 to 3 days or less. Hypodermoclysis is underutilized in the home care setting due to lack of understanding of the route and concerns about how patients would tolerate or experience this route. Advantages to hypodermoclysis include ease of initiation, minimal adverse reactions, and ability to administer a reasonable volume. Note that hypodermoclysis is a route that has been used since the 1950s and is today seeing a resurgence as it is recognized as a relatively easy, low-risk, and cost-effective method for delivery of hydration fluids in patients with mild to moderate dehydration (Caccialanza et al., 2016; Humphrey, 2011; Scales, 2011). The most commonly administered isotonic fluids include 0.9% sodium chloride and 5% dextrose in water. In an older study that included 30 long-term care residents from 24 to 90 years of age, who received SC infusions from 1 to 2 days for dehydration, all infusions were completed without adverse effects except for one incidence of local edema at the site (Walsh, 2005).

PATIENT SELECTION CONSIDERATIONS

- The patient and family are motivated and willing and capable of participating in infusion management.
- The patient is clinically stable.
  - The patient is exhibiting signs of mild to moderate dehydration; treatment of severe dehydration would not be appropriate in the home.
  - The patient is at known risk for dehydration (e.g., expected side effects with chemotherapy, and hyperemesis gravidarum).
- An appropriate infusion route is selected.
  - Short peripheral IV catheters, midline peripheral catheters, or PICCs are common VADs that may be used for fluid replacement.
  - SC route is appropriate for older adults or other adults with limited venous access and no existing VAD.
- The home environment is safe, clean, with adequate refrigeration space, and the patient has ready access to a telephone.
- Reimbursement is verified.
  - Private third-party payers vary in coverage.

COMPREHENSIVE CARE, ASSESSMENT, AND MONITORING

Plan for Home Care and Visit Frequency

- Schedule home visits to coincide with the time of fluid administration with the infusion pharmacy and the patient. This may involve two visits per day to coincide with initiating and discontinuing the infusion.
- Continued frequency of home visits depends on patient condition, degree of independence with infusion care, and ongoing needs.

Fluid and Electrolyte Administration

- Ensure that orders include name(s) of fluid, volume, route, duration of treatment, rate and method of administration.
  - The infusion rate for fluid replacement varies widely. For patients without any cardiac or other conditions that increase the risk of fluid overload, the infusion rate may be high (e.g., infuse a liter of fluid over 3 to 4 hours). For older adults and others at risk, slow infusion rates are appropriate.
  - Safe concentrations for electrolyte replacement should be addressed with the pharmacist and physician. For example, high concentrations of potassium in excess of 40 mEq/L require electrocardiographic monitoring and are thus inappropriate for home administration (Phillips & Gorski, 2014).
- Hypodermoclysis: Refer to Chapter 6 for site assessment and device placement, infusion guidelines, and monitoring for complications.
  - Isotonic fluids are usually administered. Common solutions used include 0.9% sodium chloride and 5% dextrose in water. Potassium chloride 20 to 40 mmol/L can be added to the solution (Gorski et al., 2016, p. S123; Scales, 2011).
  - The infusion is set up the same as an IV administration. A standard administration set is used for hypodermoclysis, and gravity administration is recommended (Scales, 2011), although infusion pumps may also be used (Caccialanza et al., 2016).
  - Up to 1,500 mL over 24 hours (~ 60 mL/hr) can be delivered to a single SC site, and up to 3 L may be given using two different sites. A simple Y tubing connected to the IV administration set can deliver fluids via two different sites simultaneously (Parker & Henderson, 2010). There are also specially designed SC infusion sets that allow for simultaneous infusion via two or more sites.
- IV fluid administration:
  - Electronic infusion devices used most often for rate control to reduce the risk for fluid volume overload due to too rapid infusion.

Assessment and Monitoring

- Vital signs and other expected routine assessment parameters appropriate to patient's condition (e.g., wounds, pain management, and lung sounds)

- Monitor for signs of excess fluid volume (i.e., overload)
- Monitor for improvement in symptoms associated with dehydration
- Hypodermoclysis: Complications are generally minor and may include itching or burning at the site, erythema, induration, pain, leaking, bleeding, infection, and tissue slough. Some edema is expected with hypodermoclysis but will subside as the fluid is absorbed and generally causes no discomfort. Should large and/or progressive edema occur, the infusion rate is in excess of absorption and the infusion rate should be slowed down or the infusion stopped (Caccialanza et al., 2016)
- Appearance of VAD site, patency of VAD, and any subjective complaints (e.g., pain during infusion)
- Laboratory studies as pertinent
- Overall response to home therapy

Psychosocial Considerations

- Uncertainty related to disease process and outcome of treatment
- Financial concerns

PATIENT EDUCATION: KEY POINTS

- Sorting/organizing all supplies and equipment
- Importance of handwashing
- Concept of aseptic technique
- Preparing the IV bag/container and tubing; setting up and programming the infusion pump; troubleshooting, and infusion pump safety as appropriate to goals of infusion therapy (i.e., self-care)
- VAD-related care
- Self-monitoring symptoms (e.g., signs/symptoms of fluid overload, and VAD site) including signs and symptoms to report to the nurse/physician

TEST YOUR KNOWLEDGE

1. The percentage of total body water in older adults is about:
   a. 40%
   b. 50%

   c. 60%

   d. 70%

2. Signs/symptoms of moderate dehydration include:

   a. Inability to sweat

   b. Hypotension

   c. Fever

   d. Low urine output

3. A laboratory indicator described by some as the gold standard used to diagnose dehydration is:

   a. Serum osmolality

   b. BUN

   c. Serum creatinine

   d. Urinalysis results

4. What types of fluids are administered via hyperdermoclysis?

   a. Hypotonic

   b. Hypertonic

   c. Isotonic

   d. Dextrose-free

ANSWERS

1. a

2. d

3. a

4. c

References

Armstrong, L. E., Kavouras, S. A., Walsh, N. P., & Roberts, W. O. (2016). Diagnosing dehydration? Blend evidence with clinical observations. *Current Opinion in Clinical Nutrition and Metabolic Care, 19*, 434–438.

Caccialanza, R., Constans, T., Cotogni, P., Zaloga, G. P., & Pontes-Arruda, A. (2016). Subcutaneous infusion of fluids for hydration or nutrition: A review. *Journal of Parenteral and Enteral Nutrition.* [Epub ahead of print]. doi:10.1177/0148607116676593

Gorski, L. A., Hadaway, L., Hagle, M., McGoldrick, M., Orr, M., & Doellman, D. (2016). Infusion therapy standards of practice. *Journal of Infusion Nursing, 39*(1S), S1–S159.

Hooper, L., Abdelhamid, A., Attreed, N. J., Campbell, W. W., Channell, A. M., Chassagne, P., . . . Hunter, P. (2015). Clinical symptoms, signs and tests for identification of impending and current water-loss dehydration in older people (review). *Cochrane Database of Systematic Reviews*, Issue 4, Art. No: CD009647. doi:10.1002/14651858.CD009647.pub2

Humphrey, P. (2011). Hypodermoclysis: An alternative to IV infusion therapy. *Nursing, 41*(11), 16–17.

Konrad, D., Roberts, S., Corrigan, M. L., Hamilton, C., Steiger, E., & Kirby, D. F. (2016). Treating dehydration at home avoids healthcare costs associated with emergency department visits and hospital readmissions for adult patients receiving home parenteral support. *Nutrition in Clinical Practice.* [Epub ahead of print]. doi:10.1177/0884533616673347

Mentes, J. C. (2012). Nursing standard of practice protocol: Managing oral hydration. Retrieved from https://consultgeri.org/geriatric-topics/hydration -management

Miller, H. J. (2015). Dehydration in the older adult. *Journal of Gerontological Nursing, 41*(9), 8–13.

Morley, J. E. (2015). Dehydration, hypernatremia, and hyponatremia. *Clinical Geriatric Medicine, 31*, 389–399.

Parker, M., & Henderson, K. (2010). Alternative infusion access devices. In M. Alexander, A. Corrigan, L. Gorski, J. Hankins, & R. Perucca (Eds.), *Infusion nursing: An evidence-based practice* (3rd ed., pp. 516–524). St. Louis, MO: Saunders/Elsevier.

Phillips, L., & Gorski, L. A. (2014). *Manual of IV therapeutics: Evidence-based practice for infusion therapy.* Philadelphia, PA: F.A. Davis.

Scales, K. (2011). Use of hypodermoclysis to manage dehydration. *Nursing Older People, 23*(5), 16–22.

Walsh, G. (2005). Hypodermoclysis: An alternate method for rehydration in long-term care. *Journal of Infusion Nursing, 28*(2), 123–129.

9

Antimicrobial Therapy

Antimicrobial drug administration is the most common home infusion therapy and is used to treat infections in both adult and pediatric patient populations. Given a safe home setting, an appropriate vascular access device (VAD), and a clinically stable patient responding to therapy, most antimicrobial drugs can be safely administered at home. Most often patients or their caregivers are taught how to independently administer their infusions. Studies suggest that there is no evidence of higher rates of VAD complications or worse clinical outcomes for those who self-administer as compared to when health care providers (usually nurses) administer the infusions (Barr, Semple, & Seaton, 2012; Bhavan, Brown, & Haley, 2015). A wide range of infectious diseases may be treated at home. Common diagnoses include cellulitis, osteomylelitis, bacterial endocarditis, infections associated with cystic fibrosis, and central nervous system–related infections. Increasingly, patients are treated at home without prior hospitalization.

After reading this chapter, the reader will be able to:

- Summarize patient selection criteria
- Describe key aspects of intravenous (IV) antibiotic administration
- Summarize components of comprehensive care, assessment, and monitoring

PATIENT SELECTION CONSIDERATIONS

- The patient and family are motivated and willing and capable of participating in self-infusion management.
  - In general, the goal in home administration of antimicrobial medications is patient/caregiver independence with self-infusion.
  - For patients who require a relatively short course of IV therapy or if there are functional or cognitive limitations that impact ability to learn infusion procedures, the home care nurse may provide the home infusions depending upon available reimbursement. Other options for infusion delivery include outpatient facilities, physician offices, ambulatory infusion centers, or long-term care facilities.
- The patient is clinically stable.
  - The patient's infectious disease is responding to antimicrobial treatment.
  - The patient is tolerating the antimicrobial drug without significant reactions or reactions are managed with adjunctive treatments (e.g., amphotericin B–related chills and fever managed with premedication with acetaminophen and diphenhydramine).
  - First dose issues: When possible, first doses are best administered in a controlled environment with access to emergency medical equipment and medications. Guidelines from the United Kingdom state that the first doses may be administered in the patient's home if administered by a person competent and equipped to identify and manage anaphylaxis (Chapman et al., 2012). There were no anaphylactic reactions in a study of 770 patients who received antimicrobials at home with 25 different medications including first doses (Dobson, Boyle, & Loewenthal, 2004). The Infusion Nurses Society (Gorski, Hadaway, Hagle, McGoldrick, Meyer, & Orr, 2016) provides guidance for first doses in the home setting as follows:
    - The home care agency has a first dose protocol.
    - There is reasonable access to emergency services should a severe reaction occur.
    - Patient is alert, cooperative, and able to respond appropriately.
    - Informed consent—patient understands the potential risks of a first dose.

- Medications are available in the home and there are orders for their use in the treatment of anaphylaxis/severe drug reaction.
  - An example of an adult anaphylaxis protocol is 0.2 to 0.5 mL of 1:1,000 epinephrine intramuscularly (IM) and 50 mg diphenhydramine IV in the event of signs/symptoms.
    - The patient has no history of severe allergic reactions.
    - The nurse administers the first dose and observes the patient for a minimum of 30 minutes after infusion completion.
- An appropriate VAD is in place to administer antimicrobial therapy.
  - Short peripheral IV catheters, midline peripheral catheters, or peripherally inserted central catheters (PICCs) are common VADs for antimicrobial administration. The decision is based upon a number of factors including anticipated duration of therapy, infusate characteristics, and the patient's vascular access as discussed in Chapters 4 and 5.
- The home environment is safe, clean, with adequate refrigeration space, and the patient has ready access to a telephone.
  - Antimicrobial drugs and related supplies are generally delivered to patient homes on a weekly basis. Many antimicrobial drugs require storage in the refrigerator.
- Reimbursement is verified.
  - Private third-party payers vary in coverage.
  - Certain antimicrobial drugs may be covered under the durable medical equipment benefit for external infusion pumps under Part B of the Medicare program. These include acyclovir, foscarnet, ganciclovir, and amphotericin B.

ANTIMICROBIAL MEDICATIONS

Antimicrobial medications include the use of antibacterial, antiviral, antifungal, and antiprotozoal drugs. Antibacterial drug selection is based on attaining bacteriostatic (slowing down bacterial growth) or bacteriocidal (destroying bacteria) activity at the site of the infection. Antiviral drugs, such as ganciclovir and acyclovir, slow down viral multiplication by incorporating into the virus' DNA.

Antibiotic medications are classified based upon the similarity of their chemical structures and mechanisms of action. A helpful summary of antibiotic classifications is found in a clinical article by Percival (2017). Because antibiotics are so commonly administered, home care nurses must have a sound understanding of indications, expected dosage, and adverse reactions. Antibiotics are classified as follows:

- Beta-lactams, which include the subgroups of penicillins, cephalosporins, and the carbapenems (e.g., imipenem, meropenum, ertapenum).
- Glycopeptides, which include only vancomycin in the United States. Vancomycin is commonly home administered, used to treat gram-positive organisms including methicillin resistant staphyloccoccus aureus (MRSA), has a narrow therapeutic index, requires serum concentration monitoring, and is nephrotoxic.
- Cyclic lipopeptides, which include only daptomycin, which is also commonly administered at home. It is also used to treat gram-positive organisms such as MRSA and vancomycin-resistant enterococci (VRE). Myopathy is an adverse effect with weekly monitoring of creatine phosphokinase (CPK) levels recommended.
- Lipoglycopeptides are the newest class of gram-positive antibiotics. They include telavancin, dalbavancin, and oritavancin.
- Aminoglycosides include gentamicin, tobramycin, and amikacin and are used to treat gram-negative bacteria. Because of their narrow therapeutic index, serum concentrations must be carefully monitored. Toxicities include nephro- and ototoxicity. (Percival, 2017)

In a recent descriptive study of 1,461 courses of outpatient antimicrobial therapy (OPAT) in the home, the most common antimicrobials administered were vancomycin (36%), piperacillin/tazobactam (13%), ceftriaxone, ertapenem, and daptomycin (Shrestha et al., 2016).

Antimicrobial Lock Technique

For patients who require long-term infusion therapy, the CVAD becomes the patient's "lifeline." Efforts are aimed at CVAD preservation whenever possible. In patients who experience repeated episodes of catheter-related bloodstream infection (CR-BSI), antimicrobial lock technique has been used to successfully eradicate infections and avoid catheter removal. Antimicrobial locking solutions may be used for both infection prophylaxis and for treatment of CVAD-related infection. The technique includes the use of a highly concentrated antibiotic or an antiseptic agent instilled into the internal lumen of a central venous access device and is allowed to dwell for a prescribed duration of time (e.g., 12 hours per day in between intermittent infusions). Antiseptic solutions include ethanol, taurolidine, and citrate among others. The catheter manufacturer's directions for use of ethanol should be reviewed as ethanol can cause damage to CVADs made of polyurethane. Antimicrobial locking is used in patients with long-term CVADs, patients with a history of multiple CR-BSIs, and high-risk populations (Gorski, Hadaway, Hagle, McGoldrick, Orr, & Doellman, 2016, p. S79). The procedure includes instillation of the antimicrobial solution in a volume approximately equal to the catheter lumen and allowing it to dwell for the prescribed duration of time. It is important that the antimicrobial locking solution is aspirated at the end of the locking period to reduce the risk of adverse effects including development of antimicrobial resistance (Gorski, Hadaway, Hagle, McGoldrick, Orr, & Doellman, 2016, p. S79). Antimicrobial lock technique may be administered in conjunction with systemic IV antibiotic therapy.

COMPREHENSIVE CARE, ASSESSMENT, AND MONITORING

Plan for Home Care and Visit Frequency

- Schedule home visits to coincide with the time of drug administration with the infusion pharmacy and the patient.
  - For patients continuing antimicrobial therapy started in another health care setting, ensure consistent serum drug levels by continuing previous dosing schedule (e.g., doses at 8 a.m. and 8 p.m. in hospital continue at home).
  - Adjustments in times for home administration may be made to better accommodate the patient's schedule. Gradual changes (1–2 hours per day) in time of dose may be required; consult with pharmacist.
  - To promote consistent serum drug levels and optimal antimicrobial treatment, each dose is given within 1 hour of the scheduled infusion time.
- Decrease frequency of home visits as patient/caregiver learn to self-administer the infusion and as patient assessment is stable.

- Continued frequency of home visits depends upon patient condition, degree of independence with infusion care, and frequency of physician office visits:
  - For patient independent with antimicrobial drug infusions, weekly (or more often) home visits for CVAD site care and assessment (e.g., PICC care) are usually indicated.

Drug Administration

- Ensure that orders include name(s) of drug, dosage, route, duration of treatment, rate, and method of administration.
  - Some antimicrobial drugs may also have orders for premedications (e.g., acetaminophen and diphenhydramine prior to the infusion of amphotericin B).
- Administration methods vary based upon issues such as frequency of administration, infusion rate, drug stability in solution, safety concerns, and reimbursement. They are discussed in detail in Chapter 7.
  - Gravity drip is a common and cost-effective administration method.
  - Elastomeric pumps are also commonly used. They are easy to teach to patients and caregivers but more costly compared to other methods, especially as the number of doses per day increases.
  - IV push administration may be appropriate for certain antimicrobials such as some cephalosporins.
  - Syringe pumps may be used but are generally limited to lower volume infusions.
  - Bedside electronic infusion devices (EIDs) are used less often but offer rate control when higher volumes are required (e.g., vancomycin and amphotericin B) for intermittent doses and are usually less costly than an ambulatory pump.
  - Ambulatory EIDs are often used with antimicrobial drugs given three or more times per day (e.g., penicillin G every 6 hours).
- Ensure that an order for anaphylaxis treatment is included when first doses are administered in the home setting and that ordered drugs are available in the patient's home.
- Compare and verify orders on infusion container/cassette to physician's order.
- Verify infusion parameters on EID (e.g., rate and reservoir volume) prior to starting pump.

- Verify patient identification.
- Verify patency of CVAD including presence of free-flowing blood return.
- Use "SASH" technique when administering antimicrobial medications to establish venous access device patency and to avoid heparin–drug incompatibilities (if heparinized VAD; **S**aline, **A**dminister medication, **S**aline, **H**eparin).
  - Note that a few drugs are incompatible with normal saline (e.g., amphotericin B and quinupristin/dalfopristin) and dextrose 5% in water (D5W) is used to flush the venous access device before and after infusion (Gahart, Nazareno, & Ortega, 2016). In this case, follow the D5W flush with normal saline; dextrose should not reside in the catheter lumen as it provides nutrients for biofilm growth (Gorski, Hadaway, Hagle, McGoldrick, Orr, & Doellman, 2016, p. S77).

Assessment and Monitoring

- Vital signs and other expected routine assessment parameters appropriate to patient's condition (e.g., wounds, pain management and lung sounds)
- Appearance of VAD site, patency of VAD, and any subjective complaints (e.g., pain during infusion)
- Laboratory studies as pertinent
- Overall response to home therapy
- Potential side effects or toxicities of antimicrobial drug(s). Consult a drug resource for information related to the specific antimicrobial drug administered including dosage guidelines, adverse drug reactions, drug interactions, and monitoring parameters (e.g., Gahart et al., 2016). Table 9.1 summarizes *some* common reactions and nursing interventions related to antimicrobial medications.

Psychosocial Considerations

- Explore and address potential concerns and issues throughout the course of home care.
- Specific issues may include:
  - Uncertainty related to disease process and outcome of treatment
  - Financial concerns

Table 9.1

Adverse Reaction Monitoring: Home Antimicrobial Administration

Adverse reaction/side effect	Monitor for signs/symptoms (s/s)	Nursing actions/patient education
Allergic reactions Increased risk in patients with history of penicillin allergy	Mild/localized symptoms—rash, itching, erythema, and edema Severe/sudden—anaphylaxis reactions with s/s of pruritus, urticaria, angioedema, bronchospasm, hypotension, and tachycardia	■ When first doses administered, ensure emergency medications in home with orders for use, monitor carefully for s/s, and initiate anaphylactic protocol in the event of occurrence (e.g., stop infusion immediately; call emergency services i.e. 911, administer emergency medications as ordered and monitor vital signs) ■ Teach patient s/s to report ■ Emphasize continued need to monitor and report when independent with infusion administration (reactions may occur late in treatment) ■ For mild symptoms, some physicians may treat with diphenhydramine; in other cases, the drug will be discontinued/changed
"Red man" or "red neck" syndrome Associated with vancomycin	Red, flushing maculpapular rash of the trunk, neck, face, and chest	■ Caused by a release of histamine when vancomycin is administered too rapidly ■ Stop infusion in the presence of symptoms; in most cases, resume infusion at slower rate when symptoms subside ■ Administer over at least 1 hour; some patients may require longer infusions ■ Diphenhydramine may be used as a premedication ■ Infusion pump recommended

Nephrotoxicity Associated with aminoglycosides, vancomycin, amphotericin B, acyclovir, ganciclovir, cidofovir Especially those with impaired renal function; *elderly, children,* and those receiving other nephrotoxic drugs	Increased serum drug levels Increased serum creatinine Decreased urine output	■ Teach patient about risk of nephrotoxicity and to report symptoms such as any decrease in urine output ■ Maintain timing of antibiotics to ensure consistency of serum levels ■ Teach to maintain adequate hydration ■ Monitor laboratory findings; ensure that MD is notified ■ Ensure accuracy of drug levels; trough levels just prior to drug administration; peak levels generally 1 hour postinfusion ■ Anticipate decreased doses and/or less frequent administration for patients with decreased renal function ■ Anticipate adjustments in dosage and frequency with increase in creatinine, drug levels
Ototoxicity Associated with aminoglycosides and vancomycin Especially those with impaired renal function, who have prolonged treatment, taking other ototoxic drugs (e.g., furosemide) *May be irreversible*	Loss of high-frequency sound perception, tinnitus, dizziness, nausea, and vomiting	■ Teach patients about risk, s/s, and importance of immediate reporting ■ Maintain timing of antibiotics to ensure consistency of serum levels ■ Report any s/s to MD immediately

(continued)

Chapter **9** Antimicrobial Therapy

Table 9.1

Adverse Reaction Monitoring: Home Antimicrobial Administration (*continued*)

Adverse reaction/side effect	Monitor for signs/symptoms (s/s)	Nursing actions/patient education
Diarrhea Particularly with clindamycin, and certain cephalosporins (e.g., ceftriaxone, cefoperaxone, and cefepime)		■ Teach patient to report ■ Maintain adequate hydration ■ Instruct regarding treatment as ordered per MD ■ Secure lab specimen for *Clostridium difficile* as ordered
Superinfection Appearance of clinical or microbiological evidence of a new infection during the treatment of a primary one Associated with broad spectrum antibiotics (e.g., cephalosporins, tetracyclines, and aminoglycosides)	Recurrent fever, diarrhea, sore mouth, and vaginal itching/discharge	■ Monitor for and instruct patient in s/s to report

PATIENT EDUCATION: KEY POINTS

- Sorting/organizing all supplies and equipment
- Importance of handwashing
- Concept of aseptic technique
- Preparing the IV bag/container and tubing
- Setting up and programming the infusion pump; troubleshooting, and infusion pump safety
- VAD-related care
- Drug actions and side effects
- Potential complications and actions to take
- Self-monitoring symptoms such as changes in infectious process (e.g., wound changes)
- Signs and symptoms to report to the physician

TEST YOUR KNOWLEDGE

1. The first dose of an IV antimicrobial drug may be administered under the following circumstance:
   a. The physician states that there are no risks and no special precautions
   b. The first dose may be given only via a peripheral catheter
   c. The nurse administers the dose and observes the patient postinfusion for at least 45 minutes
   d. There are orders for use of emergency medications available in the home
2. Bacteriostatic antimicrobial drugs:
   a. Kill the bacteria causing the infection
   b. Slow down the growth of bacteria causing the infection
   c. Both kill and slow down bacterial growth
   d. Slow down viral growth
3. Agents used for antimicrobial lock technique include:
   a. Low antibiotic concentrations
   b. Ethanol
   c. High heparin concentrations
   d. Dextrose
4. Red neck syndrome associated with vancomycin infusion is:
   a. An anaphylactic reaction
   b. A histamine release reaction
   c. An expected side effect
   d. A risk especially with elderly patients

5. While many medications may affect renal function, an antimicrobial drug associated with a high risk for nephrotoxicity is:
   a. Ertapenem
   b. Cefazolin
   c. Gentamicin
   d. Daptomycin

6. Ototoxicity is:
   a. A reversible and minor side effect
   b. Associated with the cephalosporin drug group
   c. Irreversible
   d. Associated with ertapenem and daptomycin

ANSWERS

1. d
2. b
3. b
4. b
5. c
6. c

References

Barr, D. A., Semple, L., & Seaton, R. A. (2012). Self-administration of outpatient parenteral antibiotic therapy and risk of catheter-related adverse events: A retrospective cohort study. *European Journal of Clinical Microbiology and Infectious Diseases, 31*, 2611–2619.

Bhavan, K. P., Brown, L. S., & Haley, R. W. (2015). Self-administered outpatient antimicrobial infusion by uninsured patients discharged from a safety-net hospital: A propensity-score-balanced retrospective cohort study. *PLOS Medicine, 12*(12), e1001922. doi:10.1371/journal.pmed.1001922

Chapman, A. L. N., Seaton, R. A., Cooper, M. A., Hedderwick, S., Goodall, V., Reed, C., . . . Nathwani, D. (2012). Good practice recommendations for outpatient parenteral antimicrobial therapy (OPAT) in adults in the UK: A consensus statement. *Journal of Antimicrobial Chemotherapy, 67*, 1053–1062.

Dobson, P. M., Boyle, M., & Loewenthal, M. (2004). Intravenous antibiotic therapy and allergic drug reactions. *Journal of Infusion Nursing, 27*, 425–430.

Gahart, B. L., Nazareno, A. R., & Ortega, M. Q. (2016). *Gahart's 2016 intravenous medications: A handbook for nurses and health professionals* (32nd ed.). St. Louis, MO: Elsevier.

Gorski, L. A., Hadaway, L., Hagle, M., McGoldrick, M., Meyer, B., & Orr, M. (2016). *Policies and procedures for infusion therapy.* Norwood, MA: Infusion Nurses Society.

Gorski, L. A., Hadaway, L., Hagle, M., McGoldrick, M., Orr, M., & Doellman, D. (2016). Infusion therapy standards of practice. *Journal of Infusion Nursing, 39*(1S), S1–S159.

Percival, K. M. (2017). Antibiotic classification and indication review for the infusion nurse. *Journal of Infusion Nursing, 40*(1), 55–63.

Shrestha, N. K., Shrestha, J., Everett, A., Carroll, D., Gordon, D., Butler, R., & Rehm, S. J. (2016). Vascular access complications during outpatient parenteral antimicrobial therapy at home: A retrospective cohort study. *Journal of Antimicrobial Therapy, 71*(2), 506–512.

10

Home Parenteral Nutrition

Parenteral nutrition is the intravenous (IV) administration of nutrients via the venous system. In the past, IV nutrition was referred to as "hyperalimentation" or "total parenteral nutrition" but the current terminology is simply parenteral nutrition (PN), and in the case of home care, home PN (HPN). Administration of HPN is a well-accepted home infusion therapy. HPN may be a short-term therapy for some patients; for example, those who require a period of bowel rest as with pancreatitis, presence of fistulas, exacerbation of inflammatory bowel disease, or with disorders such as hyperemesis gravidarum. It may be a long or even lifetime therapy for patients with disorders such as short bowel syndrome, motility disorders (e.g., scleroderma), or malignancies. Pediatric indications for HPN are similar to adults including bowel rest, malabsorption, and motility disorders. PN is a complex infusion therapy that requires considerable patient education and patient monitoring. The American Society for Parenteral and Enteral Nutrition (A.S.P.E.N.), and more recently the European Society for Clinical Nutrition and Metabolism (ESPEN) provide standards and guidelines providing direction for HPN administration (e.g., Ayers et al., 2014; Boulatta et al., 2014; Durfee et al., 2014; Pironi et al., 2016).

After reading this chapter, the reader will be able to:

- Summarize patient selection criteria
- Describe key aspects of PN administration

- Summarize components of comprehensive care, assessment, and monitoring
- Prepare a plan for patient education

UNDERSTANDING PN: AN OVERVIEW

Components of PN Solution

The PN solution is formulated based upon a formal and individualized nutritional assessment. Nutritional requirements vary based on age, nutritional status, disease, organ function, metabolic condition, and duration of PN. Due to the high-energy needs associated with growth, fluid and caloric requirements of pediatric patients are diverse within the ages of birth to 18 years.

HPN is most often administered with the fat emulsion, dextrose, amino acids, and other additives mixed in a single container. This is called "3-in-1" or "total nutrient admixture (TNA)." Infusion administration for home patients is simplified with the use of a single container. Components of PN solution include fluid, protein, carbohydrate, fat, electrolytes, vitamins and trace minerals, and medications.

Fluid

- Basic requirements are 30 to 35 mL/kg/d.
- Fluid needs are higher when there are significant fluid losses (e.g., diarrhea and enterocutaneous fistula).

Protein

- It is required for tissue growth and repair and replacement of all body cells.
- There is no storage of protein; all protein is functional.
- It is provided in the form of synthetic amino acids, both essential and nonessential.
- Various commercial formulations and concentrations are available.

Carbohydrate

- Major function is as an energy-providing nutrient, sparing body protein.
- If not immediately used, it is stored in the liver and muscle as glycogen; when glycogen storage is exhausted, excess carbohydrate is then stored as fat.

- Needs are based on estimation of energy requirements; generally used to provide about 50% of calories in PN solution.
- It provides 4 kcal/g.

Fat

- Its primary purpose is to provide metabolic fuel and prevent essential fatty acid deficiency (EFAD); EFAD can occur in as little as 5 days without supplementation (Krzywda & Meyer, 2014).
- It is provided in the form of lipid emulsion that contains a combination of essential and nonessential fatty acids, glycerin, and phospholipids.
- It is more calorically dense providing 9 kcal/g.

Electrolytes

- Standard preparations are available in premixed formulas that include sodium, potassium, magnesium, calcium, chloride, and phosphorus.
- Additional amounts are added based on patient need determined by serum electrolyte levels.

Vitamins and Trace Elements

- Multivitamins should be a component of all PN formulas (Durfee et al., 2014).
- Multivitamin solution is added to the HPN solution just prior to initiating infusion because there is lack of long-term stability of vitamins in solution.
- Vitamin K is included in the pediatric multivitamin preparation but is not included in the standard adult multivitamin solution; must be added separately.
- Trace elements are micronutrients that are found in the body in minute amounts (Table 10.1). They include iron, iodine, zinc, copper, chromium, manganese, and selenium and molybdenum; when iron is clinically indicated, there are alternate forms available including separate infusions (Durfee et al., 2014). Iron dextran can be added to an HPN solution that does not contain fat; however, an iron dextran test is required before the initial infusion due to the risk of allergic reaction.
- Vitamin and trace element doses are adjusted as needed (Pironi et al., 2016).

Table 10.1

Trace Elements in PN Solutions

Trace element	Purpose	Signs/symptoms of deficiency
Iron	Oxygen transport	Pallor, fatigue, exertional dyspnea, tachycardia, paresthesias, and glossitis/stomatitis
Iodine	Thyroid hormone synthesis	Hypothyroidism
Copper	Involved in the action of many oxidative enzymes	Microcytic anemia, neutropenia, osteoporosis, depigmentation of hair/skin, and skeletal demineralization
Chromium	Potentiates actions of insulin	Neuropathy, insulin-resistant glucose intolerance, and hyperlipidemia
Manganese	Involved in enzyme activation	Extrapyramidal symptoms, bony abnormalities, central nervous system dysfunction, weight loss, dermatitis, nausea, vomiting, and change in hair color
Selenium	A component of various enzymes; one enzyme protects cells from lipid peroxides and free radicals	Muscle dysfunction, including cardiac and myalgias
Zinc	Most abundant trace element; needed for RNA, DNA, and protein synthesis; plays a role in wound healing	Alopecia, scaly skin, dermatitis, diarrhea, mental depression/apathy, glucose intolerance, night blindness, impaired taste/wound healing, and T-lymphocyte dysfunction
Molybdenum	Cofactor for sulfite oxidase and xanthine oxidase	Headache, night blindness, irritability, lethargy, and coma

Source: Krzywda and Meyer (2014).

PN, parenteral nutrition.

Medications

- The complexity of PN solutions increases the possibility of physiochemical interactions such as precipitation, loss of drug activity, or clumping or curdling of the solution between the drug and the solution (Rollins, 2012).
- Compatible medications that may be added to the PN include insulin, histamine receptor agonists (e.g., famotidine), and heparin. Current guidelines recommend against the addition of heparin in the PN solution as it has not been shown to decrease the risk of catheter-associated thrombosis (Boullata et al., 2014).

Fast Facts in a Nutshell

Only limited additives to any PN solution should be made outside of the compounding pharmacy. Concentrated electrolyte solutions should not be added to PN in the home and no additions to the PN solution should be made after PN administration has started.

PATIENT SELECTION CONSIDERATIONS

- The patient and family are motivated, willing, and capable of participating in self-infusion management.
  - PN is a complex therapy that must be integrated into the daily life of the patient and family. The patient or caregiver must participate in infusion administration and monitoring. With some exceptions, such as very short courses of HPN, the patient or caregiver is expected to learn how to administer PN independently.
  - Preparation for HPN varies by institution. Acute care settings with nutritional support teams provide careful patient and family evaluation and significant patient education in preparation for home care. Patients discharged from acute care settings without specialty teams may be less prepared. Home care teaching and support and the expertise of the home care clinicians become more critical.
- The patient is clinically stable prior to going home with PN.
  - Weight maintained or increased as per HPN goals
  - Stable blood chemistry levels

- Stable nutritional laboratory indicators
- No evidence of rebound hypoglycemia with discontinuation of cyclic infusions
- No adverse reactions
- The patient is stabilized on the intended home infusion regimen for PN prior to acute care discharge.
  - Patients may be converted from a continuous to a cyclic infusion at home but this requires increased monitoring for fluid volume (overload), glucose, and electrolyte imbalances as the IV rate is increased to deliver the infusion over a shorter period of time.
  - Initiating HPN without prior hospitalization is done, although infrequently. Requirements include clinical stability and capability of being educated in the home. This should be done based only on an analysis of benefits versus risks (Durfee et al., 2014). Laboratory data are obtained prior to initiation of PN. Thorough nutritional assessment and comprehensive patient and family education are required before starting HPN. Close monitoring of patient response to fluid volume continuous infusion and a decreased rate and/or concentration of infusion are also recommended.
- A central vascular access device (CVAD) is in place.
  - Patients receiving HPN may have an implanted port, a tunneled catheter, or a peripherally inserted central catheter (PICC); for long-term HPN, tunneled catheters, ports are recommended over PICCs due to higher thrombosis risk and more difficulty with self-administration with PICCs (Pironi et al., 2016).
  - Never administer HPN via a short peripheral or midline catheter because HPN solutions are irritating formulas that contain greater than 10% dextrose and/or 5% protein. Note that peripheral parenteral nutrition (PPN) may be administered by a peripheral catheter but this type of nutritional support is uncommon in home care. PPN is characterized by lower osmolarity (≤900 mOsm) and lower dextrose concentration (<10%; Boullata et al., 2014; Gorski et al., 2016).
- The home environment is safe, clean, with adequate refrigeration space, and the patient has ready access to a telephone.
  - HPN and related supplies are generally delivered to patient homes on a weekly basis. The HPN bags are stored in the refrigerator. In some cases, the home infusion pharmacy may provide a small refrigerator dedicated to PN storage.

- Reimbursement is verified.
  - Private third-party payers vary in coverage.
  - Certain diagnoses and HPN infusions may be covered under the durable medical equipment benefit under Part B of the Medicare program. Patients must meet criteria that include "permanence" interpreted as requiring HPN for at least 3 months.

COMPREHENSIVE CARE, ASSESSMENT, AND MONITORING

Plan for Home Care and Visit Frequency

- Schedule initial home visits to coincide with the initiation and the discontinuation of the (intermittent) infusion; coordinate time of infusion with patient; and allow patient input into cycle time that best fits the home routine (e.g., 12-hour infusion to run from 9 p.m. to 9 a.m. or 7 p.m. to 7 a.m.).
- Once patient/caregiver is independent with PN administration, decrease home visit frequency as appropriate.
  - Patient teaching beyond the basic techniques of infusion administration will continue.
  - Depending upon anxiety level in relation to infusion, most of teaching related to self-monitoring (e.g., potential complications) is best accomplished when patient or caregiver has mastered administration technique.
  - With subsequent home visits, schedule to coincide with infusion-related care to reassess technique, especially in relation to infection control precautions.

Fast Facts in a Nutshell

Recommendations for the pharmacy address the need for HPN labels to be readable. The label should be well-organized, in a standard format, using simple and common terms, with clear directions regarding ingredients that must be added (e.g., multivitamins). For patients with limited English proficiency, whenever possible, the directions should be in the patient's preferred language, and also in English.

PN Administration

- PN infusions may be continuous (24 hours per day) or cyclic, lasting a portion of the day (e.g., 12–16 hours per day). A cyclic administration schedule is preferred by many home care patients because they have at least some time when they are free from carrying a pump. Most patients will want to run the cyclic infusion over nighttime hours (Krzywda & Meyer, 2014). Cyclic infusions are also recommended as a strategy for reducing the risk of intestinal failure–related liver disease (Pironi et al., 2016).
- Ensure that orders include complete PN formula including additives, infusion rate and duration, and any tapering of infusion:
  - Tapered infusions mean that the infusion is gradually increased and/or decreased at the start and completion of the infusion, typically for 1 to 2 hours. Cited benefits of tapering include a decreased risk of rebound hypoglycemia, although most patients do well without a tapered infusion (i.e., consistent infusion rate over the prescribed number of hours).
  - Document the initial PN formula, and any changes, as part of the physician's orders for home care and as part of the medication profile or other appropriate form.
- Assist patient in proper storage of PN formula in refrigerator and establish safe location for additional infusion-related supplies.
- Filtration is required. For 3-in-1 PN, use a 1.2-μm filter that is bacteria/particulate retentive and air eliminating. Should a lipid emulsion be separately administered, also filter using a 1.2-μm filter in accordance with manufacturer's directions (Gorski et al., 2016).
- Hang time for PN solution is limited to 24 hours. Change administration set/filter every 24 hours. For separate administration of lipid emulsions, the hang time, and duration for changing administration set/filter is limited to 12 hours.
- Use an electronic infusion device (EID).
  - An ambulatory EID is preferred to afford patient mobility; with nighttime infusions, it provides advantages as it is easier for patient to get up at night to void.
- Ensure that label on HPN bag matches physician's order, matching all components on the label to the order.
- Inspect HPN solution visually prior to spiking the container.
  - Do not administer if past expiration date or if leaks or precipitate are noted.

- 3-in-1 HPN: Do not use if solution appears oily or separated ("cracked" solution).
- "Multichamber" PN bags separate the dextrose/amino acid from the lipid emulsion with a "bar" on the outside of the infusion bag. The bar is removed just prior to administration allowing the components of the PN to mix together. The purpose is to reduce the risk for PN solution instability or precipitation (Ayers et al., 2014).
- Verify patient identity and verify infusion parameters on infusion pump (e.g., rate, tapering period, and reservoir volume) prior to starting pump.
- Verify patency of CVAD including presence of free-flowing blood return.

Assessment and Monitoring

In relation to the administration of PN, assessment, monitoring, and potential complications can be divided into five key areas. CVAD-related complications other than infection are addressed in Chapter 5.

Infectious Complications

Patients receiving HPN have been identified as at increased risk for infection, as addressed in Chapter 3. Catheter-related bloodstream infection (CR-BSI) is considered a common and serious complication associated with long-term HPN (Buchman, Opilla, Kwasny, Diamantidis, & Okamoto, 2014). In a systematic literature review, the overall rate of CR-BSI ranged between 0.38 and 4.58 episodes/1,000 catheter days (Dreesen et al., 2013). The researchers found that Gram-positive bacteria of human skin flora caused more than half of infections and concluded that the origin of infection was multifactorial. Reduce the risk for infection as follows:

- Perform hand hygiene and aseptic technique.
- Dedicate a single lumen for HPN administration if a multilumen CVAD is in place as an infection risk reduction strategy (Ayers et al., 2014; Gorski et al., 2016).
- For patients receiving PN, blood sampling from the CVAD is not recommended due to increased risk for CR-BSI (Ayers et al., 2014; Buchman et al., 2014).
- Depending upon nature of infection/causative microorganism, patient may be treated aggressively with antibiotics, including antibiotic lock technique (addressed in Chapter 9; Gorski et al.,

2016, p. S79). Treatment is aimed at preservation of the CVAD whenever possible.

Alterations in Blood Glucose

Blood glucose levels should be checked while the patient is not receiving the (intermittent) PN infusion (levels should be normal) and during the PN infusion. Current guidelines recommend maintaining blood glucose less than 180 mg/dL during HPN infusion and normal hemoglobin A1C levels, if patient is diabetic (Pironi et al., 2016).

- Obtain blood glucose parameters from the ordering physician.
- Monitor blood glucose frequently at beginning of HPN, with any changes in insulin.
- For patients with elevated blood glucose levels, anticipate changes in the PN regimen such as lengthening the infusion time for cyclic PN, decreasing dextrose and increasing fat calories, and/or adding insulin to the solution.

Alterations in Fluid Volume Status and/or Electrolytes

Be aware that abnormalities may occur in previously stable patients in situations such as acute diarrhea, increased fistula output, or vomiting.

- Monitor for signs/symptoms (s/s) of fluid/electrolyte imbalances (Table 10.2). Anticipate routine laboratory monitoring including complete metabolic profile, complete blood count. The frequency of laboratory monitoring is based upon patient condition, often weekly at the onset. For patients who are stable on long-term HPN, monitoring may be monthly or less frequent.
- Notify physician if signs/symptoms present; check serum levels to validate.
- Anticipate changes in HPN formula; some patients may require additional IV hydration fluids.
- If converting infusion from continuous to cyclic or if decreasing infusion time period, assess patient for signs/symptoms of fluid overload as infusion rate is increased.

Alterations in Liver Function and Metabolic Bone Disease

- Know the risk factors, especially for patients on long-term PN.
- Bone disease in adults likely results from underlying disease, malabsorption, and chronic steroid use. Symptoms may include

back pain, bone pain, and fracture. Routine monitoring of bone densitometry scanning and biochemistry is recommended for long-term HPN and periodically thereafter (Pironi et al., 2016).

- Liver disease associated with HPN includes steatosis, cholestasis, and gallbladder stones (Kumpf & Gervasio, 2012). The causes are not clear but factors may include continuous dextrose infusion, EFAD, excessive lipid infusion, amino acid imbalance, toxic effects of HPN degradation products, and overgrowth of intestinal flora (Krzywda & Meyer, 2014). Periodic monitoring of liver function tests is recommended. Pediatric patients who receive long-term HPN are at high risk for associated liver disease affecting 50% to 66% of patients (Israelite, 2017). Preventative strategies include avoidance of overfeeding, cyclic HPN, limiting the dose of soybean-based lipid to less than 1 g per day, and prevention and management of sepsis (Pironi et al., 2016).

Nutrition-Related Complications

- Know the goals of HPN and include in the plan of care. Some examples include maintaining weight, increasing weight to __ pounds, achieving improved nutritional state as evidenced by increased serum albumin, closure of an enterocutaneous fistula.
- Assess indicators of nutritional status regularly including weight, skin integrity, elimination, behavioral changes (e.g., listlessness vs. alertness), mucous membranes, nail bed, oral cavity including teeth and tongue, and circulatory status (e.g., presence of edema).
- EFAD may occur in those patients who do not receive lipid emulsions as part of the PN formula. Signs/symptoms include alopecia, impaired wound healing, thrombocytopenia, dry and scaly skin, and elevated liver enzymes.
- Assess for s/s of vitamin and trace element (Table 10.2) deficiencies. Recommendations for laboratory monitoring include baseline measurements at the onset of HPN and then at least once per year (Pironi et al., 2016).

Fast Facts in a Nutshell

For pediatric patients, plotting of height, weight, and head circumference (age 3 and under) using a growth chart is essential to determine if there is any faltering of growth.

Table 10.2

Electrolyte Imbalances Associated With PN

Electrolyte	Signs/symptoms
Sodium: Excess ■ Most often associated with decreased fluid volume	Serum sodium level greater than 145 mEq/L
	Thirst, dry mucous membranes, fever, hypotension, low urine output, and poor skin turgor
Sodium: Deficiency ■ Most often associated with increased fluid volume	Serum sodium level less than 135 mEq/L
	Nausea, vomiting, muscle weakness/twitching/cramps, weight gain, and confusion
Potassium: Excess	Serum potassium level greater than 5.5 mEq/L
	Paresthesias, diarrhea/nausea, cramping, irritability, weakness, and atrial/ventricular arrhythmias
Potassium: Deficiency	Serum potassium level less than 3.5 mEq/L
	Fatigue, leg cramps, paresthesias, muscle weakness, drowsiness, nausea, vomiting, decreased bowel motility, irregular pulse, and arrhythmias
Magnesium: Excess	Serum magnesium level greater than 3 mEq/L
	Flushing, skin warmth, nausea, vomiting, drowsiness, muscle weakness, and respiratory depression
Magnesium: Deficiency	Serum magnesium level less than 1.5 mEq/L
	Paresthesias, cramps, muscle weakness, increased reflexes, positive Chvostek's and Trousseau's signs, convulsions, tachyarrhythmia, confusion, and mood changes
Calcium: Deficiency	Serum calcium level less than 8.5 mg/dL
	Numbness, tingling of fingers, toes or circumoral area, muscle cramps, positive Chvostek's and Trousseau's signs, confusion, memory changes, and convulsions
Phosphorus: Deficiency	Serum phosphate level less than 2.5 mg/dL
	Paresthesias, muscle weakness, confusion, and seizures

Note: Calcium excess and phosphorus excess states are uncommon in patients on PN.
Source: Adapted from Phillips and Gorski (2014).
PN, parenteral nutrition.

Psychosocial Considerations

Explore and address potential concerns and issues with patient and caregiver(s) throughout the course of home care. Psychosocial considerations are often considerable for the patient who is unable to eat "normally" and who requires lifelong PN. Yet, studies show little attention is also paid to these issues (Huisman-de Waal, van Achterberg, Jansen, Wanten, & Schoonhoven, 2011). In a recent qualitative study exploring the experience of adults dependent on HPN, the concept of "normalization" was a repeating and strong theme (Winkler & Smith, 2015). It is vitally important that nurses who care for patients on HPN understand the issues and the need for patients to maintain as much normality in life as possible. Specific issues may include:

- Fear and anxiety related to HN
- Loss of ability to eat
- Changes in family life/roles
- Depression
- Caregiver stress
- Body image alterations
- Financial concerns

Fast Facts in a Nutshell

The Oley Foundation is the national support and information group for patients who are on PN or enteral nutrition. Written patient educational materials, newsletters, and support group information are provided. Membership is free to patients. Finding "others who are like me" was an attribute of "normalization" in the Winkler and Smith (2015) study (the website is www.oley.org).

Gordon Meier, a former pastor, chronicles the challenges and his journey of living on HPN in his book *Taste—My New Life Without Food:*

> My doctor indicated that in all likelihood I will stay on TPN the rest of my life and implied that I will never eat again. . . . That diagnosis has caused me to have days filled with darkness and dread, but also times filled with overwhelming gratitude for my many blessings . . . The prospect of never eating again is

something that I still can't wrap my mind around, but God has poured out His grace and continues to give me endurance to live one day at a time, until I can eat again. (Meier, 2013, pp. 14–15)

PATIENT EDUCATION: KEY POINTS

- Sorting/organizing/safe storage of all supplies and equipment
- Safety precautions related to disposal of used HPN bags and supplies
- HPN infusion
  - Infection prevention including hand hygiene and aseptic technique
  - Preparing the IV bag/container and tubing
  - Mixing and adding medications (e.g., multivitamin) to the HPN bag
  - Setting up and programming the infusion pump
  - Troubleshooting, infusion pump alarms
  - CVAD-related care: Site care and assessment, flushing, and cap/valve changes
- Self-monitoring parameters such as daily weight, temperature, blood glucose, intake and output
- Signs/symptoms of potential complications/problems, actions to take, and reporting to the physician or nurse

TEST YOUR KNOWLEDGE

1. Which component of the HPN solution is required for tissue growth and repair?
   a. Carbohydrate
   b. Protein
   c. Trace elements
   d. Vitamins
2. A symptom of EFAD is:
   a. Diarrhea
   b. Anemia
   c. Dry and scaly skin
   d. Decreased liver enzymes
3. The most abundant trace element is:
   a. Iodine
   b. Selenium

      c. Zinc
      d. Iron
4. A metabolic advantage to cyclic HPN includes:
      a. Reduced risk of liver problems
      b. Reduced risk of fluid volume overload
      c. Better glucose control
      d. Reduced risk of vitamin deficiencies
5. To reduce the risk for CR-BSI, which of the following is
   recommended?
      a. Avoid the use of PICCs for HPN infusion
      b. Decrease the concentration of glucose in the HPN solution
      c. Avoid drawing blood for laboratory sampling from the CVAD
      d. Administration of continuous HPN
6. The purpose of a multichamber bag is:
      a. Reduce the risk for HPN solution instability
      b. Simplify HPN administration
      c. Decrease the risk for electrolyte imbalance
      d. Decrease loss of vitamin potency
7. Current recommendation regarding blood glucose levels is to
   maintain the level:
      a. Below 100 mg/dL
      b. Below 150 mg/dL
      c. Below 180 mg/dL
      d. Below 200 mg/dL
8. Which of the following has been cited as a failure in HPN
   management?
      a. Not addressing psychosocial issues
      b. Not identifying trace element deficiencies
      c. Not assessing nutritional status
      d. Not administering a cyclic infusion

ANSWERS

1. b
2. c
3. c
4. a
5. c
6. a
7. c
8. a

References

Ayers, P., Adams, S., Boullata, J., Gervasio, J., Holcombe, B., Kraft, M. D., . . . Worthington, P. (2014). A.S.P.E.N. parenteral nutrition safety consensus recommendations. *Journal of Parenteral and Enteral Nutrition*, *38*(3), 291–333.

Boullata, J. I., Gilbert, K., Sacks, G., Labissiere, R. J., Crill, C., Goday, P., . . . American Society for Parenteral and Enteral Nutrition. (2014). A.S.P.E.N. clinical guidelines: Parenteral nutrition ordering, order review, compounding, labeling, and dispensing. *Journal of Parenteral and Enteral Nutrition*, *38*(3), 334–377.

Buchman, A. L., Opilla, M., Kwasny, M., Diamantidis, T. G., & Okamoto, R. (2014). Risk factors for the development of catheter-related bloodstream infections in patients receiving home parenteral nutrition. *Journal of Parenteral and Enteral Nutrition*, *38*(6), 744–749.

Dreesen, M., Foulon, V., Spriet, I., Goossens, A. G., Hiele, M., De Pourcq, L., & Willems, L. (2013). Epidemiology of catheter-related infections in adult patients receiving home parenteral nutrition: A systematic review. *Clinical Nutrition*, *32*, 16–26.

Durfee, S. M., Adams, S. C., Arthur, E., Corrigan, M. L., Hammond, K., Kovacevich, D. S., . . . American Society for Parenteral and Enteral Nutrition. (2014). A.S.P.E.N. standards for nutrition support: Home and alternate site care. *Nutrition in Clinical Practice*, *29*(4), 542–555.

Gorski, L. A., Hadaway, L., Hagle, M., McGoldrick, M., Orr, M., & Doellman, D. (2016). Infusion therapy standards of practice. *Journal of Infusion Nursing*, *39*(1S), S1–S159.

Huisman-de Waal, G., van Achterberg, T., Jansen, J., Wanten, G., & Schoonhoven, L. (2011). High tech home care: Overview of professional care in patients on home parenteral nutrition and implications for nursing care. *Journal of Clinical Nursing*, *20*(15–16), 2125–2134.

Israelite, J. C. (2017). Pediatric parenteral nutrition-associated liver disease. *Journal of Infusion Nursing*, *40*(1), 51–54.

Krzywda, E., & Meyer, D. (2014). Parenteral nutrition. In M. Alexander, A. Corrigan, L. A. Gorski, & L. Phillips (Eds.), *Core curriculum for infusion nursing* (5th ed., pp. 309–355). Philadelphia, PA: Lippincott Williams & Wilkins.

Kumpf, V. J., & Gervasio, J. (2012). Complications of parenteral nutrition. In C. M. Mueller (Ed.), *The A.S.P.E.N. adult nutrition core curriculum* (2nd ed., pp. 284–297). Silver Spring, MD: American Society for Parenteral Enteral Nutrition.

Meier, G. F. (2013). *Taste—my new life without food.* (Self-published)

Phillips, L., & Gorski, L. A. (2014). *Manual of IV therapeutics: Evidence-based practice for infusion therapy.* Philadelphia, PA: F.A. Davis.

Pironi, L., Arends, J., Bozzetti, F., Cuerda, C., Gillanders, L., Jeppesen, P. B., . . . Home Artificial Nutrition and Chronic Intestinal Failure Special Interest Group of ESPEN. (2016). ESPEN guidelines on chronic intestinal failure in adults. *Clinical Nutrition*, *35*(2), 247–307.

Rollins, C. J. (2012). Drug-nutrient interactions. In C. M. Mueller (Ed.), *The A.S.P.E.N. adult nutrition core curriculum* (2nd ed., pp. 298–312). Silver Spring, MD: American Society for Parenteral Enteral Nutrition.

Winkler, M. F., & Smith, C. E. (2015). The impact of long-term home parenteral nutrition on the patient and the family: Achieving normalcy in life. *Journal of Infusion Nursing*, *38*(4), 290–300.

11

Chemotherapy Infusions

Administration of chemotherapy in the home setting varies across different regions of the country. Because of the need for close monitoring and risk of drug reactions, complex multidrug regimens are infrequently administered in the home setting. However, for patients who require longer infusions of chemotherapy drugs, home care offers a cost-effective option and a variety of advantages often expressed by health care providers and patients including decreased risk of infection in the home, ability to continue many normal activities of daily living, and participation in own care. Although not widely practiced, home administration of chemotherapy for pediatric patients may also offer advantages such as improved appetite, well-being, and ability to keep up with school work and less disruption in the family routine.

Safety is paramount when administering home chemotherapy. Because the consequences of a chemotherapy error could result in significant patient harm, chemotherapy agents are on the list of "high-alert" medications for both acute and community-based care (Institute for Safe Medication Practices [ISMP], 2011, 2014). The Oncology Nursing Society (ONS, 2015), in a position paper, asserts that only qualified clinicians administer cancer chemotherapy and biotherapy based on completion of a specialized education and competency program, and furthermore recommends an annual assessment of competency. This paper and position are supported also by the Infusion Nurses Society (INS; Gorski et al., 2016, p. S127). Safe preparation and handling of chemotherapy agents in the home is essential. The nurse must understand dose-limiting toxicities of chemotherapy drugs, expected side effects, and strategies for management. The reality is that most chemotherapy drugs are administered in outpatient settings and the home care nurse may administer only a portion of the protocol. However, in managing this patient population, the home care nurse must be well-educated in overall monitoring, side effects, and patient education. The home care nurse plays an important role in managing the physical and psychological effects of chemotherapy (White, 2015). The ONS provides online courses in chemotherapy administration, which can be found on the website www.ons.org/education.

After reading this chapter, the reader will be able to:

- Summarize patient selection criteria
- Describe key aspects of chemotherapy administration including safe practices
- Summarize components of comprehensive care, assessment, and monitoring
- Prepare a plan for patient education

OVERVIEW OF CHEMOTHERAPY

Chemotherapy drugs administered in the home setting most often are those given as an intermittent or continuous infusion. Adjuvant drugs such as those that potentiate the action of the chemotherapy agent (e.g., leucovorin with 5 fluorouracil [5-FU]) or rescue agents may be part of the regimen (e.g., mesna to prevent hemorrhagic cystis). Other therapies may be administered in conjunction with the chemotherapy such as hydration fluids, antiemetic or anti-infective drugs, and/or hematopoietic growth factors (e.g., filgrastim).

The basic mechanism of chemotherapy is to interrupt the synthesis of DNA, disrupting cell division and causing cell death. Chemotherapy drugs may exert their action during a specific phase of the cell or may exert their effect in all phases of the cell cycle. *Cell cycle–specific* drugs include drugs classified as antimetabolites (e.g., 5-FU), vinca alkaloids, and a variety of miscellaneous agents. *Cell cycle–nonspecific* drugs include drugs classified as alkylating agents, antitumor antibiotics (e.g., doxorubicin), hormonal agents, and nitrosureas. These drugs act on cells that are not going through the cell division stage. Because chemotherapy agents do not distinguish cancer cells from normal cells, those cells that are frequently dividing are affected including those in the bone marrow, gastrointestinal tract, mucosa, gonads, and hair follicles. Side effects resulting from damage to these cells include myelosuppression, nausea, vomiting, diarrhea, mucositis, infertility, and hair loss (Czaplewski & Vizcarra, 2014).

The drug 5-FU is commonly administered as a home infusion for patients. Based on the protocol for the patient's cancer diagnosis, infusions may be over 22 to 48 hours every 1 to 3 weeks or as a continuous infusion lasting 5 to 8 weeks (Chavis-Parker, 2015). There is scarce reporting of other home-administered chemotherapy drugs. Additional chemotherapy drugs that have been home administered, based on this author's experience, are presented in Table 11.1. Consult a drug resource (e.g., Gahart, Nazareno, & Ortega, 2016) or other chemotherapy reference for information about other chemotherapy drugs and for specifics of drug actions, dosing, and additional information. Cancer care and treatment also include numerous biological agents that are administered as infusions such as monoclonal antibodies, fusion proteins, interleukins, and immunoglobulins. There is scarce data regarding the administration of biologicals for cancer treatment in the home setting. The risk of severe reactions is often a limiting factor. For this reason, this chapter is limited to only chemotherapy cancer treatment. Immunoglobulin therapy, which may be administered in the treatment of cancer, may be home-administered and is addressed in Chapter 14.

PATIENT SELECTION CONSIDERATIONS

- The patient and family are motivated, willing, and capable of participating in self-infusion management.
  - Chemotherapy infusions may be continuous or long intermittent infusions (hours) and are delivered via a central vascular access device (CVAD) using an infusion pump. This requires at least some level of patient or caregiver participation in infusion administration, venous access device–related care, and monitoring.
- The patient is clinically stable prior to initiating chemotherapy.
  - Nutritional status is adequate and the patient is able to tolerate adequate food and fluid intake.
  - Elimination status includes adequate bowel and urine elimination.
  - Recent hematologic and renal function laboratory results are checked. General guidelines for administering chemotherapy include:
    - Serum creatinine and blood urea nitrogen (BUN) are within normal limits.

Table 11.1

Selected Chemotherapy Drugs

Drug classification	Drug	Common indications	Side effects/toxicities	Additional information
Antimetabolite, cell cycle specific	Cytarabine (ARA-C, Cytosar-U)	AML, ALL, CML, Hodgkin's and non-Hodgkin's lymphoma, and CNS leukemia	Myelosuppression, nausea, vomiting, anorexia, fever, mucositis, diarrhea, liver/renal dysfunction, and photophobia	■ Given as IV or subcutaneous infusion ■ Nadir—4–10 days ■ Oral care instructions
	Floxuridine (FUDR)	Gastrointestinal tract adenocarcinoma with liver metastasis	Liver toxicity, gastritis, dermatitis, mucositis, and diarrhea	■ Given as a hepatic intra-arterial infusion
	Fluorouracil (5-FU)	Cancer of the colon, breast, liver, ovary, pancreas, rectum, stomach, esophagus, and head and neck	Mild myelosuppression, nausea, vomiting, diarrhea (dose limiting), mucositis, photosensitivity, dry skin, and hand and foot syndrome	■ Instruct patient to wear sunscreen ■ Report watery diarrhea, changes in skin (extremities), mouth sores ■ Leucovorin potentiates antitumor activity of 5-FU—increases risk and severity of SE
	Methotrexate	Non-Hodgkin's lymphoma, ALL, AML, breast, lung, head and neck cancers, and CNS metastasis	Myelosuppression, mucositis, nausea, vomiting, photosensitivity, and liver/renal toxicity	■ Leucovorin used to prevent toxicity with high doses; protects kidneys and prevents lethal bone marrow suppression and stomatitis

Alkylating agent	Cyclophosphamide (Cytoxan)	Ewing's sarcoma, Burkitt's tumor, breast, ovarian cancers, multiple myeloma, lymphoma, neuroblastoma	Hemorrhagic cystitis, myelosuppression, nausea and vomiting, and alopecia	▪ Instruct patient to take multivitamin with folic acid ▪ Use sunscreen, eye protection ▪ Good oral care
				▪ Hydration essential to reduce risk for hemorrhagic cystitis ▪ Empty bladder frequently ▪ Nadir—7–14 days
	Ifosfamide (IFEX)	Lung, testicular cancer, non-Hodgkin's lymphoma, and sarcoma	Hemorrhagic cystitis, nausea, vomiting, alopecia, myelosuppression, and neurotoxicity	▪ Mesna is always given as a rescue agent ▪ Mesna can be mixed with ifosfamide in same IV bag
Vinca alkaloid	Vincristine (Oncovin)	ALL, Hodgkin's and non-Hodgkin's lymphoma, breast cancer, rhabdomyosarcoma, and Wilms tumor	Neurotoxicity (dose limiting) including peripheral neuropathy, constipation, paralytic ileus, numbness, weakness, cramping, foot drop, and also alopecia	▪ *Vesicant drug;* if extravasation occurs, apply heat to area 15–20 minutes QID for the first 24–48 hours ▪ Notify physician ▪ Nadir—5–10 days ▪ Bowel regimen

(continued)

Table 11.1

Selected Chemotherapy Drugs (continued)

Drug classification	Drug	Common indications	Side effects/toxicities	Additional information
Antitumor antibiotics; cell cycle nonspecific	Doxorubicin (Adriamycin)	Breast, ovary, prostate, stomach, thyroid cancers, small cell lung cancer, squamous cell cancer of head and neck, Hodgkin's and non-Hodgkin's lymphoma, ALL, and multiple sclerosis	Myelosuppression, nausea and vomiting, alopecia, cardiac toxicity (dose limiting), hyperuricemia, and photosensitivity	■ *Vesicant drug:* if extravasation occurs, apply cold/ice pack to area 15–20 minutes QID for the first 24–48 hours; notify physician immediately; dexrazoxane is the antidote that is administered as a daily infusion for 3 days ■ Lifetime cumulative dose of 550 mg/m² (450 mg/m² if prior chest irradiation or concomitant cyclophosphamide therapy) ■ Turns urine reddish orange that disappears ~24 hours after infusion
	Mitoxantrone (Novantrone)	Breast cancer, AML, multiple sclerosis	Myelosuppression, arrhythmias, and cardiac toxicity	■ IV push and intermittent infusion ■ Turns urine blue green for 1–2 days after infusion ■ May turn sclera bluish
Other	Cladribine	Hairy cell leukemia	Myelosuppression, hypersensitivity, and rash	■ May be given as a 7-day infusion ■ Nadir—7–10 days

ALL, acute lymphocytic leukemia; AML, acute myeloid leukemia; CML, chronic myeloid leukemia; CNS, central nervous system; IV, intravenous; SE, side effect; QID,

❑ Platelets are more than 100,000.
❑ Absolute neutrophil count (ANC)* is more than 1,500.

> *Even if the white blood cell (WBC) count is normal, neutropenia can exist. Calculate the ANC as follows:
>
> Multiply the total WBC by the total percentage of neutrophils (polys [or segs] + bands)
>
> Example:
>
> WBC is 2,000, polys are 45%, bands are 3%
>
> $ANC = 2,000 \times (0.45 + 0.03) = 960$

- The patient has previously received the chemotherapy drug without reaction.
- A CVAD is in place.
  - Patients may have an implanted port (very common), a tunneled catheter, or a peripherally inserted central catheter (PICC).
  - Peripheral intravenous (IV) or midline catheters are not used to administer continuous vesicant infusions (Gorski et al., 2016).
- The home environment is safe, clean, with adequate refrigeration space, and the patient has ready access to a telephone.
- Reimbursement is verified.
  - Private third-party payers vary in coverage.
  - Certain diagnoses and continuous chemotherapy infusions may be covered under the durable medical equipment benefit for external infusion pumps under Part B of the Medicare program.

COMPREHENSIVE CARE, ASSESSMENT, AND MONITORING

Plan for Home Care and Visit Frequency

- Schedule initial home visits to coincide with the initiation and the discontinuation of the (intermittent) infusion.
- Follow up by telephone 2 to 3 days after infusion starts to identify if there are any problems or side effects (e.g., nausea, vomiting, and diarrhea).

- Schedule a home visit or telephone call during nadir period to assess for any signs/symptoms of infection.
- Coordinate overall plan for home care with physician office/outpatient chemotherapy clinic.

Safety and Home Chemotherapy

Drug Preparation and Storage

- Chemotherapy drugs are prepared in the infusion pharmacy and delivered to the home ready for administration.
- IV drug reservoirs/bags are delivered "preprimed" from the infusion pharmacy.
- Store drug, supplies, and cytotoxic waste container in an area safe from children and pets.

Drug Administration

- Wear personal protective equipment (PPE; e.g., chemotherapy gloves and impermeable gown).
- Use a plastic-backed pad on a clean surface to set up supplies and drug reservoir/pump.
- Use all luer-lock connections.
- Discard all used supplies that have had contact with the chemotherapy (e.g., gloves and tubings) in the cytotoxic waste container.

Spills

- A "spill kit" is provided by the infusion pharmacy.
- The spill kit includes PPE, absorbent sheets/materials for containing the spill, and plastic bag for disposal with label for contaminated items.
- Instruct the patient and caregiver in how to use the spill kit should any leaks occur.
- A chemotherapy spill should be reported as an agency occurrence.

Chemotherapy Administration

- Coordinate the time of the infusion with the referring physician, infusion pharmacy, and the patient. Certain chemotherapy protocols are very specific in terms of timing. The infusion chemotherapy administered by the home care nurse is often part of a protocol that is administered in the outpatient clinic.
- A written order from a physician or licensed provider with appropriate credentialing is needed for the administration of all

chemotherapeutic agents. Verbal and telephone orders are not acceptable except in the instance of discontinuing a chemotherapy medication.

- The drug order includes patient's name, drug name(s), dosage/m^2 or dose per unit body weight or dose for an area under the concentration–time curve (AUC), and/or total dose, frequency, and route.
- Orders may also include premedications (e.g., antiemetic) and/or plan for hydration, if needed.
- Dosage information should be verified by two professionals (e.g., registered nurse and infusion pharmacist).
- Ensure that orders for extravasation and anaphylaxis treatment (if applicable) are included if vesicant drugs or first doses are administered.
- Check that laboratory values are within acceptable parameters for the drug to be administered.
- Recalculate body surface area (BSA) and drug dosage; websites are available for calculation (e.g., www-users.med.cornell .edu/~spon/picu/calc/bsacalc.htm).
- Compare order on infusion container to physician's order and verify infusion parameters on pump (e.g., rate and reservoir volume) prior to starting pump.
  - Consider a double-check system such as having the home care nurse call the pharmacist while in the home and read the infusion pump parameters. There are reported cases of patient death and hospitalization due to pump parameter errors resulting in overdoses of 5-FU (Ewen, Combs, Popelas, & Faraone, 2012; ISMP Canada, 2007). Based on such medication safety issues, the use of elastomeric devices (in contrast to a programmable infusion pump) for 5-FU was evaluated ($N = 574$ home care patients) and was found to be a safe administration method (Broadhurst, 2012).
- Use appropriate PPE.
- Verify patency of CVAD including presence of free-flowing blood return.

Assessment and Monitoring

Immediate Complications of Chemotherapy Administration

Extravasation
Extravasation is defined as the inadvertent administration of vesicant medication or solution into the surrounding tissue instead of into the

intended vascular pathway (Gorski et al., 2016). Vesicant drugs are those capable of causing tissue injury and are highlighted in Table 11.1.

- Extravasation can occur when drugs are administered through a CVAD.
- Causes of CVAD-related extravasation include incomplete port needle insertion, dislodged port needle, catheter separation from body of port, damaged catheter (e.g., hole in tunneled catheter under the skin), backtracking of medication along catheter into subcutaneous tissue.
- Prevention of extravasation:
  - Use a noncoring needle to access port that is long enough to touch bottom of port and can be stabilized and secured to the skin.
  - Assess for signs of venous thrombosis prior to starting infusion. If present, notify physician and ensure that patient has radiographic flow study prior to CVAD use.
  - Ensure that there is a free-flowing blood return prior to administration of the vesicant. Never start a vesicant infusion in the home without obtaining a blood return.
  - Ask the patient if there is any pain, burning, or stinging as the CVAD is flushed with saline and assess for any swelling in the area. Other signs of concern include shoulder pain and ringing in ears during flushing. If present, do not initiate chemotherapy; contact physician to discuss need for radiographic study of catheter placement/flow.
  - Stabilize port needle and pump tubing to avoid tension or "pulling" at needle insertion site.
  - Teach patient about risks and preventive actions (Patient Education: Key Points).
  - Refer to Chapters 4 and 5 for management of extravasation.

Anaphylaxis
- Avoid first doses of chemotherapy drugs in the home.
- If first dose is given, ensure presence of and orders for emergency drugs (e.g., epinephrine and diphenhydramine) and remain in the home for 20 to 30 minutes after initiation of infusion to monitor for any reactions.
- Instruct patient and family in actions to take should a severe reaction occur (call 911).

Side Effect Management

Bone Marrow Suppression

The risk is greatest during the drug's nadir period, the time when the blood count reaches its lowest point. For most chemotherapy agents, this occurs about 7 to 10 days after drug administration.

- Monitor WBC (ANC), hemoglobin, and platelet count.
- Monitor for signs/symptoms of infection, bleeding (including occult bleeding and headache), and anemia.
- Monitor temperature. Be aware that if patient is neutropenic, fever (≥100.4) is the most reliable and often only indicator of infection (ONS, 2001). A fever needs to be reported to the physician immediately.
- Instruct patients in good handwashing and hygiene including oral and perineal care, and bleeding precautions.
- Instruct patients to avoid persons with contagious illnesses, especially during nadir period.
- Anticipate potential treatment with hematopoietic growth factor either at home or in the clinic.

Gastrointestinal Side Effects

- Monitor for nausea, vomiting, diarrhea, mucositis, stomatitis, and anorexia.
- Administer and/or provide patient education regarding supportive treatments (e.g., antiemetic and antidiarrheal medications).
- Instruct patient in eating strategies including: small frequent meals; how to increase fluid intake; eating high calorie, high protein foods; and taking nutritional supplements.
- Instruct patient to avoid irritants such as alcohol and tobacco.
- Instruct in regular oral care, avoid commercial mouthwashes, and use soft toothbrush.
- Notify physician for persistent nausea and vomiting beyond 24 hours, diarrhea lasting 2 to 3 days, fever, mouth/rectal pain or sores, and inability to eat.

Integumentary Side Effects

- These include alopecia and dermatitis ("hand and foot syndrome," especially associated with 5-FU infusion).
- Instruct patient to use mild shampoo, decrease frequency of hair care, avoid permanents and other hair processing, and protect scalp from heat and cold.

- Instruct patient regarding protection of hands and feet during very cold or hot weather conditions and use protection if touching heated cooking utensils or containers from the freezer.
- Provide patient with information about resources (e.g., American Cancer Society's Look Good, Feel Better program; www.cancer.org/treatment/supportprogramsservices/look-good-feel-better).
- When significant hair loss is anticipated, encourage patients to match hair color/style with wig before hair loss occurs (if desired).
- Report signs of dermatitis such as scaling, peeling, numbness or tingling, redness, and pain; ensure supportive treatments such as pain control, cold compresses, elevation, ointments, and lotions.

Neurological Side Effects
- Understand the dose-limiting toxicity of vinca alkaloids, cisplatin, and taxol.
- Monitor for paresthesias, constipation, paralytic ileus, muscle flaccidity, foot drop; report occurrences to physician.
- Be aware that constipation is often minimized by patients.
- Instruct patient to increase fluid intake, maintain fiber in diet, and take stool softeners/stimulants (Polovich, Whitford, & Olsen, 2014).

Psychosocial Considerations

Explore and address potential concerns and issues throughout the course of home care.
- Specific issues may include:
  - Patient/family goals and expected results
  - Quality of life issues
  - Changes in family roles
  - Maintaining activities of daily living
  - Uncertainties of treatment outcomes
  - Financial concerns

PATIENT EDUCATION: KEY POINTS

- Sorting/organizing all supplies and equipment
- Safety precautions related to storage of chemotherapy drug, supplies, and cytotoxic waste container

- For patients who are involved with some level of administration:
  - Concept of aseptic technique
  - Setting up and programming the infusion pump
  - Troubleshooting
- CVAD-related care
- Patient self-monitoring as indicated (e.g., reportable side effects/ adverse drug reactions, CVAD/peripheral site, and laboratory work schedule)
- Signs and symptoms to report to the physician or nurse
- Safe handling and disposal of contaminated materials
  - Laundry: Wear gloves while handling contaminated laundry, wash separately from other laundry using hot water and detergent.
  - Family members should wear gloves when handling body fluids or soiled linens.
  - Refrain from close sexual contact during the first 48 hours after chemotherapy/cytotoxic agents is completed.
  - Precautions are in effect during a minimum of 48 hours after the chemotherapy agent is competed (Polovich et al., 2014).
- High-risk infusions: Continuous vesicant infusion via a CVAD; instruct patient in:
  - Signs and symptoms to report: Pain, burning, stinging, soreness at port or catheter site
  - Checking the dressing at least daily
  - Importance of calling the agency immediately and stopping the pump if any wetness, leaking, redness, or swelling is noted at the port/catheter site
  - Careful dressing and undressing to avoid pulling at port/ catheter site; women should make sure that bra straps do not rub over catheter exit site/port area
- Resource: National Cancer Institute: Access to many helpful patient-teaching publications (cancer.gov/cancerinfo/treatment)

TEST YOUR KNOWLEDGE

1. The following drug is considered a vesicant:
   a. Cladribine
   b. Cytoxan
   c. Doxorubicin
   d. Methotrexate

2. The patient is receiving a vincristine infusion and the needle dislodges from the patient's implanted port; some drug has extravasated into the tissue; anticipate which of the following critical steps is helpful to manage this extravasation:
   a. Immediately place ice over the area
   b. Use warm packs over the area
   c. Transfer within 6 hours for patient to receive the antidote drug dexrazoxane
   d. Instruct to immediately take an anti-inflammatory drug such as ibuprofen
3. Patients should be instructed to handle body waste/excretions carefully for at least 48 hours. This includes:
   a. Wear gloves while handling contaminated laundry
   b. Wash linens that have not had contact with chemotherapy with bleach
   c. Do not allow any other family members to use the same toilet
   d. Do not touch any other family members
4. Using the BSA calculator website given in this chapter, or the BSA calculator website of your choice, calculate the BSA for a patient who is 5'7" tall and weighs 155 lb.
   a. 1.36 m^2
   b. 1.81 m^2
   c. 1.25 m^2
   d. 1.73 m^2
5. Side effects associated with 5-FU include:
   a. Myelosuppression, mucositis, photosensitivity
   b. Hyperuricemia, myelosuppression, mucositis
   c. Myelosuppression, photosensitivity, renal toxicity
   d. Mucositis, impotence, photosensitivity
6. Calculate the ANC: the WBC is 1,500; the percentage of neutrophils (polys + bands) is 45%.
   a. 720
   b. 675
   c. 500
   d. 680

ANSWERS

1. c
2. b
3. a

4. b
5. a
6. b

References

Broadhurst, D. (2012). Transition to an elastomeric infusion pump in home care: An evidence-based approach. *Journal of Infusion Nursing, 35*(3), 143–151.

Chavis-Parker, P. (2015). Safe chemotherapy in the home environment. *Home Healthcare Now, 33*(5), 246–251.

Czaplewski, L. M., & Vizcarra, C. (2014). Antineoplastic and biologic therapy. In M. Alexander, A. Corrigan, L. A. Gorski, & L. Phillips (Eds.), *Core curriculum for infusion nursing* (5th ed., pp. 258–308). Philadelphia, PA: Lippincott Williams & Wilkins.

Ewen, B. M., Combs, R., Popelas, C., & Faraone, G. M. (2012). Chemotherapy in home care: One team's performance improvement journey towards reducing medication errors. *Home Healthcare Nurse, 30*(1), 28–37.

Gahart, B. L., Nazareno, A. R., & Ortega, M. Q. (2016). *Gahart's 2016 intravenous medications: A handbook for nurses and health professionals* (32nd ed.). St. Louis, MO: Elsevier.

Gorski, L. A., Hadaway, L., Hagle, M., McGoldrick, M., Orr, M., & Doellman, D. (2016). Infusion therapy standards of practice. *Journal of Infusion Nursing, 39*(1S), S1–S159.

Institute for Safe Medication Practices. (2011). ISMP list of high-alert medications in acute care settings. Retrieved from http://ismp.org/communityRx/tools/highAlert-community.pdf

Institute for Safe Medication Practices. (2014). ISMP list of high-alert medications in community/ambulatory healthcare. Retrieved from http://ismp.org/Tools/institutionalhighAlert.asp

Institute for Safe Medication Practices Canada. (2007). Fluorouracil incident root cause: Follow-up analysis. Retrieved from https://www.ismp-canada.org/download/reports/FluorouracilIncidentMay2007.pdf

Oncology Nursing Society. (2015). Education of the nurse who administers and cares for the individual receiving chemotherapy and biotherapy. Retrieved from https://www.ons.org/advocacy-policy/positions/education/chemotherapy-biotherapy

Polovich, M., Whitford, J., & Olsen, M. (Eds.). (2014). *Chemotherapy and biotherapy guidelines and recommendations for practice* (3rd ed.). Pittsburgh, PA: Oncology Nursing Society.

White, K. (2015). Supporting individuals receiving chemotherapy in their home. *Australian Nurse Midwife, 23*(6), 47.

12

Infusion Pain Management

Infusion pain management includes the administration of opioid analgesics via the subcutaneous (SC), intravenous (IV), or intraspinal route. Additional medications, such as low doses of anesthetic agents, may be used with intraspinal infusions. In the home care setting, the patient population includes primarily those with chronic pain, either cancer related or chronic pain of a nonmalignant nature. Patients may be under traditional home care or in home hospice. Infusion pain management is never the first choice. It is more complicated for patients and families, more costly, and associated with risks such as catheter-related complications. Before proceeding to an infusion pain management strategy, the current pain management plan is always carefully evaluated. Some questions to ask before deciding on an infusion route include:

- Were appropriate analgesics given according to the World Health Organization (WHO) cancer pain ladder for adults? These include appropriate use of oral opioid and nonsteroidal anti-inflammatory drugs (NSAIDs), and use of adjuvant drugs as appropriate such as an anticonvulsant for neuropathic pain (WHO, 2016). The pain ladder could be applied to noncancer pain as well.
- Was the pattern of taking pain medicines appropriate (e.g., around the clock)?
- Were other noninvasive routes evaluated (e.g., transdermal)?
- Was there an adequate trial of each intervention?
- Were nonpharmacologic interventions included in the pain management plan?

- Does the patient have: persistent gastrointestinal side effects (e.g., nausea and vomiting) associated with high doses of oral opioids; inability to take oral medications (e.g., dysphagia and obstruction); need for rapid titration of analgesics?

Pain management, and infusion pain management in particular, is complex requiring significant knowledge on the part of the home care nurse. This chapter provides an overview of key issues.

After reading this chapter, the reader will be able to:

- Summarize patient selection criteria
- Describe key aspects of analgesic administration
- Summarize components of comprehensive care, assessment, and monitoring
- Prepare a plan for patient education

UNDERSTANDING PAIN MANAGEMENT: INFUSION ROUTE OPTIONS

SC Route

The SC route represents the standard of care for managing moderate to severe pain when the oral and rectal routes are not available or appropriate (Weissman, 2015a). Drugs that may be administered SC include morphine, hydromorphone, fentanyl, and sufentanil as either bolus doses or continuous SC infusion. Although clinicians believe that cachectic, febrile, or hypotensive patients will have difficulty with SC absorption, there are no data to support this (Weissman, 2015a). Infusion rates of 3 to 5 mL per hour are usually considered acceptable (Gorski et al., 2016). Some patients may tolerate higher infusion rates. Patient-controlled analgesia (PCA) can be used in conjunction with a basal rate. Information specific to SC infusion is included in Chapter 6.

Advantages include:
- Readily available; as vascular access is not required
- Less costly and less complicated than IV route
- Easy to initiate in the home setting
- Patient/family can learn to rotate sites

Limitations:

- More difficult to titrate
- Must use concentrated drug to keep infusion rates low

IV Route

IV infusions may be continuous, intermittent bolus, and/or PCA. Information specific to vascular access devices (VADs), care and maintenance, and potential complications are included in Chapters 4 and 5. The IV route allows for rapid titration of dose to achieve pain control.

Intraspinal Route

The intraspinal route allows for delivery of analgesic and adjuvant medications (e.g., anesthetics) via the epidural or intrathecal route. Intraspinal infusions may be used in carefully evaluated patients who have not achieved pain relief despite escalating analgesic doses or who have experienced excessive systemic side effects. There is less central nervous system (CNS) depression associated with intraspinal administration. Continuous infusions are most common in home care patients. PCA may be used with epidural catheters (Gordon & Schroeder, 2015). With epidural administration, the drug must pass through the dura mater to gain access to the cerebrospinal fluid (CSF; see Chapter 6). With intrathecal administration, the drug is administered directly into the CSF where it is immediately able to bind to opiate receptor sites in the dorsal horn, located all along the spinal cord. Pain impulses are intercepted before they are transmitted to the brain. Intrathecal drug doses are approximately 1/10th the dosage of an epidural infusion.

Once the drug passes into the CSF, drug flows in two directions: primarily to the brain (rostral flow) and passively toward the base of the spine (minimal). Drug absorption is affected by:

- Lipid solubility—lipid-soluble drugs (e.g., fentanyl) penetrate dura rapidly, have a more rapid onset of action, a shorter duration, have limited spread therefore effect is mainly in the area of catheter tip placement; water-soluble drugs (morphine) take longer to diffuse, have a longer duration, are more slowly cleared, and have a broader spread of analgesic effect
- Molecular weight and volume—higher volume may have a wider effect
- Specific receptor affinities (Sterns & Brant, 2015)

Advantages to intraspinal pain management include less systemic effects, less drug requirement, and improved pain control/quality of life in patients unable to achieve pain control via less invasive methods. Limitations include higher cost, a more complex therapy requiring patient willingness, ability to manage, and, because of potential neurotoxicity, drugs must be preservative free. Information specific to epidural and intrathecal catheter placement, care and maintenance, and potential complications are addressed in Chapter 6. Refer to Table 12.1 for a list of analgesic medications used for infusion pain management.

Pediatrics and Infusion Pain Management

Home-administered opioid infusions can be administered in pediatric patients. Although there is limited research, a recent study documented the need for PCA opioid infusions for children during end-of-life and in advanced disease (Mherekumombe & Collins, 2015). This study from Australia identified 33 pediatric patients with diagnoses including metastatic bone disease, severe abdominal pain, and severe headaches. The most common infusion drugs administered were hydromorphone (more than 50%), fentanyl, morphine, and methadone with side effects that included itching, sedation, nausea, and urinary retention. The most common infusion route was via a central VAD (CVAD) and four patients received SC infusions. For 97% of the patients, the opioid infusions were continued at home until death.

PATIENT SELECTION CONSIDERATIONS

- The patient and family are motivated, willing, and capable of participating in self-infusion management.
  - Infusion analgesics are a continuous infusion administered using an infusion pump. This requires at least some level of patient or caregiver participation in infusion administration and monitoring.
- There is a responsible family member or caregiver available and willing to participate in patient care and monitoring.
  - The caregiver is available to troubleshoot problems in the event of adverse drug reactions, infusion pump problems, or deterioration in condition.
- The patient is clinically stable on the intended analgesic infusion prior to hospital discharge and subsequent home care admission.
  - Patients taking oral or transdermal opioid drugs may be converted to a SC or IV analgesic infusion in the home

Table 12.1

Analgesic Medications Used in Infusion Pain Management

Medication	Selected characteristics	Infusion route	Route specific: additional information
Morphine	■ Most often, drug of choice for infusion pain management due to extensive experience/research ■ Rapid onset of action (30–60 minutes) ■ Short half-life (2–4 hours)	■ SC ■ IV ■ Intraspinal (must be preservative free)	■ Intraspinal: morphine is water-soluble drug; slower movement through CSF results in longer duration of action (up to 24 hours) and slower clearance
Hydromorphone	■ More potent analgesic than morphine ■ Rapid onset of action (5 minutes) and short half-life (2–3 hours) ■ Shorter duration (3–4 hours) than morphine and less drug accumulation; may be better choice with older patients	■ SC ■ IV ■ Intraspinal (must be preservative free)	■ Because drug is more concentrated, is a good choice for subcutaneous infusions ■ More lipid soluble than morphine, therefore less rostral spread
Fentanyl	■ Rapid onset (5–15 minutes), shorter duration (1–4 hours) due to lipid solubility	■ In home care, used primarily with intraspinal infusions (must be preservative free)	■ Continuous intraspinal infusion preferred to intermittent boluses due to short duration ■ Limited rostral spread therefore effect is mainly in the area of catheter tip placement

(continued)

Table 12.1

Analgesic Medications Used in Infusion Pain Management (*continued*)

Medication	Selected characteristics	Infusion route	Route specific: additional information
Anesthetic agents	■ Low doses; block nerve fibers that carry pain with minimal sensory and motor effect ■ Goal is to provide analgesia, not anesthesia ■ Most often bupivacaine and ropivacaine ■ Moderate to fast acting (5–20 minutes) ■ Duration of action up to 12 hours	■ Intraspinal	■ May be used in conjunction with opioids and decrease opioid doses required ■ Signs of systemic toxicity include tinnitus, metallic taste, slow speech, irritability, twitching, seizures, circumoral tingling and numbness, and dysrhythmias
Clonidine	■ Usual use in hypertension; is a centrally acting α2-adrenoreceptor agonist ■ Used in intraspinal pain management for treatment of chronic neuropathic pain; thought to bind to α2-receptors located in dorsal horn near opioid receptors	■ Intraspinal (must be preservative free	■ Often used in conjunction with morphine or anesthetic agents ■ Side effects include sedation, dry mouth, hypotension, and bradycardia
Baclofen	■ Used primarily for spasticity; also found to be an effective intrathecal analgesic in chronic pain when other medications have failed/tolerance to intrathecal morphine	■ Intraspinal	■ Side effects include hypotonia, sedation, constipation, erectile dysfunction, loss of sphincter control, and respiratory depression

CSF, cerebrospinal fluid; IV, intravenous; SC, subcutaneous.

Sources: Gahart, Nazareno, and Ortega (2016); Stearns and Brant (2010)

setting; however, this requires a knowledgeable and committed patient and family. Oral or transdermal doses are converted to an equianalgesic infusion dose.

- ❑ Frequent assessment and ongoing monitoring of pain control and side effects by the nurse, and by the patient/family, are required when IV/SC analgesics are initiated in the home.

Fast Facts in a Nutshell

The Palliative Care Network of Wisconsin is the home of "Fast Facts for Palliative Care." There are hundreds of concise, referenced, and easy-to-read guidelines including many related to pain management. Opioid conversion guides are available. An app is available for smart phones. The website is www.mypcnow.org/fast-facts.

- For IV infusions, an appropriate infusion device is in place to administer infusion therapy.
  - A short peripheral IV catheter is not indicated for chronic infusion pain management due to ongoing risk of dislodgement and interruptions in pain control.
  - A midline peripheral might be selected for infusion pain management when the duration of expected need is about 1 month or less.
  - For long-term needs, a CVAD such as a peripherally inserted central catheter (PICC), subcutaneously tunneled CVAD, or implanted port is appropriate.
  - Consider the possibility of SC analgesic infusion as preferred over IV as discussed previously.
- The home environment is safe, clean, with adequate refrigeration space, and the patient has ready access to a telephone.
  - Analgesic drugs and related supplies are generally delivered to the patient home on a weekly basis. Some drugs may require storage in the refrigerator.
- Reimbursement is verified.
  - Private third-party payers vary in coverage.
  - Continuous infusion of SC, IV, and epidural opioids may be covered under the durable medical equipment benefit for external infusion pumps under Part B of the Medicare program.

COMPREHENSIVE CARE, ASSESSMENT, AND MONITORING

Plan for Home Care and Visit Frequency

- The frequency of ongoing home visits is based on various factors: degree of pain control, level of patient and family coping, and patient educational needs.
- Schedule home visits minimally to coincide with the time of drug reservoir/administration set changes (frequency varies; 3–7 days).
- The home care nurse provides infusion care in terms of changing drug reservoir or, depending on family situation, this may be taught to a competent caregiver.
- Recommend telephone follow-up between home visits to assess pain control as needed.

Analgesic Administration

- Ensure that orders include name of analgesic drug(s)/concentration, dosage per hour (called "basal rate"; usually a range allowing titration), bolus dose (about half the basal rate) and frequency/lock out period, and infusion route.
- A programmable electronic infusion pump with patient lock out (prevents ability to alter infusion rate/program) is required.
- Compare and verify analgesic orders to physician's order.
- Verify patient identification and verify infusion rate and other parameters on pump.

Fast Facts in a Nutshell

In acute care settings, an independent double check by two clinicians is often required as opioids are considered "high-alert" medications (Institute for Safe Medication Practices [ISMP], 2011). There is risk in home care. A particularly high-risk situation is when the drug concentration is increased, such as with SC infusions to reduce the hourly infusion rate/volume. Although it may be unrealistic to send two clinicians to a home with every drug reservoir change, one solution is to have the home care nurse call the pharmacist while in the home and read the infusion pump parameters.

- Titrate infusion, within physician orders for dosage range, to achieve pain control.
  - Monitor for increase in side effects with increase in dose.
  - Obtain order for increased dose range as appropriate.

Assessment and Monitoring

The patient receiving infusion pain management is monitored for adequacy of pain relief and for medication side effects.

Level of Pain Control

- Patient's self-report of pain level. Use of a pain-rating scale is recommended (e.g., 0–10 for pediatric patients—Faces Scale).
  - Ask patient about not only during time of home visit but at various times of day, during rest and activity; aggravating and relieving factors.
  - Evaluate response to bolus doses, if used
  - Assess patient satisfaction with pain; level of pain in relation to the patient's goal for pain control—(e.g., patient goal of "3" on 0–10 scale). The patient's goal for pain should be established at the beginning of home care and reevaluated at periodic intervals.
- Add up the amount of opioid analgesics used over a time period (e.g., 24 hours), including basal and bolus and increase based on severity of pain. Although there is a lack of clear data to guide any increases in analgesia, when an increase is less than 25%, patients do not notice a change in analgesia. Some general guidelines for patients who are tolerating the opioid well with no or minimal sedation include (Weissman, 2015b):
  - For ongoing mild to moderate pain, increase by 25% to 50%, irrespective of starting dose.
  - For ongoing moderate to severe pain, increase opioid doses by 50% to 100%, irrespective of starting dose. For example, a patient receives 10 mg per hour of morphine, which equals 240 mg per 24 hours. A 50% increase would be 360 mg per 24 hours or 15 mg per hour. Critical to effective pain management are the competency of the home infusion nurse in understanding pain management concepts and patient assessment as well as collaboration among the interprofessional team.
- Assess for any use/effectiveness of nonpharmacologic methods (e.g., massage, heat, cold, relaxation, and imagery).

Opioid side effects

- Constipation
  - Opioid-induced constipation (OIC) affects 45% to 90% of patients causing significant morbidity (Badke & Rosielle, 2015). This expected side effect is due to decreased gastrointestinal motility, inhibition of mucosal electrolyte and fluid transport, and interference with the defecation reflex. It is a side effect for which patients do not develop tolerance.
  - Stimulant laxatives are recommended (e.g., senna and bisacodyl). Although recommended starting doses for these medications are low, patients with OIC require higher doses. At the onset of regular opioid use, stimulant laxatives should be prescribed. Up to 12 tablets of senna or up to nine tablets of bisacodyl may be safely used (Badke & Rosielle, 2015). A stool softener alone is not effective. Osmotic laxatives (e.g., polyethylene glycol) are also used.
  - Increasing fluid intake, dietary roughage, and activity may be additional recommendations depending upon the patient's clinical situation. However, these interventions alone do not deal with the etiology of OIC.
- Sedation
  - Usually occurs within first 1 to 3 days of opioid infusion and with significant increase in dosage
  - Tolerance develops over time—days to weeks
  - Caffeine or stimulant drugs may be used
  - Sedation effect may be increased if other sedating drugs are used (e.g., muscle relaxants)
  - May respond to decrease in dosage/frequency/another opioid drug or, if all attempts fail, may be indication to attempt intraspinal pain management
  - Sudden increase in drowsiness in patients receiving epidural infusion could be caused by catheter migration into blood vessel or intrathecal space
  - Other factors also contribute to sedation such as lack of sleep from uncontrolled pain
  - Naloxone, including specific orders for use, may be kept in the home for use as needed

Fast Facts in a Nutshell

Monitor sedation. If excessive sedation is prevented, respiratory depression is prevented because more opioid is needed to cause respiratory depression than sedation.

- Nausea
  - May be due to opioid effect on chemoreceptor trigger zone in the brain, decreased GI motility, or effect on vestibular nerve
  - Usually occurs within first 1 to 3 days of opioid infusion and with increase in dosage; titrate doses slowly
  - Usually decreases over time
  - Antiemetic drugs, motility drugs, and motion sickness medications may be used
- Pruritus
  - Common with intraspinal opioid infusion, especially morphine. May be due to opioid interacting with the opiate receptors in the dorsal horn versus release of histamine (Simpson, 2010; Sterns & Brant, 2010)
  - Tends to decrease over time
  - Diphenhydramine and low doses of naloxone may be attempted
  - Cool compresses may help
- Urinary retention
  - Associated with intraspinal analgesic infusion (opioids and anesthetic agents)
  - Tolerance often develops; straight catheterization may be needed; rarely, patients may require an indwelling urinary catheter (Stearns & Brant, 2010)
  - Assess for bladder distention, voiding patterns, and urine output

Psychosocial Considerations

- Uncertainty related to disease process and outcome of treatment
- Reluctance to report pain/cultural implications
- End-of-life issues
- Family/caregiver sense of helplessness/caregiver burden
- Misconceptions and fears (e.g., addiction)
- Impact on lifestyle
- Financial concerns

PATIENT EDUCATION: KEY POINTS

- Medication actions and side effects
- Potential side effects and actions to take
- Nonpharmacologic interventions
- The infusion procedure
- VAD-related care
- Signs and symptoms to report
- Keeping a log or record of pain control is helpful; patient or caregiver records pain rating, use of bolus dose, effectiveness, and side effects
- A pain management resource
  - City of Hope—includes many publications and patient educational material that can be downloaded. The website is www.cityofhope.org.

Fast Facts in a Nutshell

The American Pain Society is a professional organization with links to many other pain resources. The website is www.ampainsoc.org.

TEST YOUR KNOWLEDGE

1. Which infusion route represents the "standard of care" for managing moderate to severe pain when the oral or rectal route is not appropriate?
   a. Intrathecal
   b. Epidural
   c. IV
   d. SC
2. A limitation to using the SC route includes a patient who:
   a. Is cachexic
   b. Is hypotensive
   c. Requires high drug doses
   d. Is hypertensive
3. What would be the most appropriate type of VAD for a patient who requires long-term IV analgesia?
   a. Peripheral catheter
   b. Midline catheter

   c. PICC

   d. Nontunneled CVAD

4. Rostral flow refers to:

   a. CSF flow to the brain

   b. CSF flow to the base of the spine

   c. Poor drug absorption

   d. Lipid solubility

5. Which statement is true about the side effect of pruritus?

   a. It is associated most often with intraspinal opioid infusion, especially morphine

   b. It is thought to be due to migration of the opioid from the intrathecal space into the bloodstream

   c. It may require an increase in opioid rate

   d. The best intervention is warm compresses

6. Which symptom might indicate systemic toxicity of an intraspinally administered anesthetic?

   a. Dry mouth

   b. Sedation

   c. Metallic taste

   d. Constipation

ANSWERS

1. d
2. c
3. c
4. a
5. a
6. c

References

Badke, A., & Rosielle, D. A. (2015). Fast facts and concepts #294: Opioid-induced constipation part I: Established management strategies. Retrieved from http://www.mypcnow.org/blank-shc3m

Gahart, B. L., Nazareno, A. R., & Ortega, M. Q. (2016). *Gahart's 2016 intravenous medications: A handbook for nurses and health professionals* (32nd ed.). St. Louis, MO: Elsevier.

Gordon, D., & Schroeder, M. (2015). Fast facts and concepts #85: Epidural analgesia. Retrieved from http://www.mypcnow.org/blank-rqvax

Gorski, L. A., Hadaway, L., Hagle, M., McGoldrick, M., Orr, M., & Doellman, D. (2016). Infusion therapy standards of practice. *Journal of Infusion Nursing, 39*(1S), S1–S159.

Institute for Safe Medication Practices. (2011). ISMP list of high-alert medications in acute care settings. Retrieved from http://ismp.org/communityRx/tools/highAlert-community.pdf

Mherekumombe, M. F., & Collins, J. J. (2015). Patient-controlled analgesia for children at home. *Journal of Pain and Symptom Management, 49*(5), 923–927.

Simpson, M. H. (2010). Pain management. In M. Alexander, A. Corrigan, L. A. Gorski, J. Hankins, & R. Perucca (Eds.), *Infusion nursing: An evidence-based approach* (3rd ed., pp. 372–390). St. Louis, MO: Saunders/Elsevier.

Stearns, C. K., & Brant, J. M. (2010). Intraspinal access and medication administration. In M. Alexander, A. Corrigan, L. A. Gorski, J. Hankins, & R. Perucca (Eds.), *Infusion nursing: An evidence-based approach* (3rd ed., pp. 535–539). St. Louis, MO: Saunders/Elsevier.

Weissman, D. E. (2015a). Fast facts and concepts #28: Subcutaneous opioid infusions. Retrieved from http://www.mypcnow.org/blank-d5l0b

Weissman, D. E. (2015b). Fast facts and concepts #20: Opioid dose escalation. Retrieved from http://www.mypcnow.org/blank-it0kw

World Health Organization. (2016). WHO's cancer pain ladder for adults. Retrieved from http://www.who.int/cancer/palliative/painladder/en

13

Cardiac Infusion Therapy

Heart failure (HF) is a prevalent diagnosis among home care patients and is a costly condition associated with both high morbidity and mortality. As the U.S. population ages and as the risk of HF increases with age, it is predicted that the number of HF cases in the United States will increase from about 5 million in 2012 to over 8 million by 2030 (Heidenreich et al., 2013). The trajectory of HF consists of exacerbations followed by periods of stability and, as disease exacerbations increase, HF worsens and may require more aggressive treatment to manage and control HF symptoms. In terms of home infusion therapies, diuretic therapy, such as periodic infusions of a loop diuretic, and positive inotropic drugs may be administered for symptom management in advanced HF, to reduce hospitalizations and improve functional status (Katz, Waters, Hollis, & Chang, 2015). Defined as drugs that increase cardiac contractility, the most commonly home-administered inotropes are dobutamine and milrinone (Katz et al., 2015; Lyons & Carey, 2013).

Cardiac infusion therapies may be administered in home care and home hospice settings and clearly, a great deal of home infusion therapy for patients with HF is considered palliative (Ciuksza, Hebert, & Sokos, 2015; Katz et al., 2015). However, while the majority of cardiac infusion therapy is among the older, chronically ill adult population, infusions are also home administered to both adults and children as a bridge to a specific cardiac intervention, such as transplantation or placement of a left ventricular assist device (LVAD; Birnbaum et al., 2015; Hashim et al., 2015).

After reading this chapter, the reader will be able to:

- Summarize patient selection criteria
- Identify the most common infusion medications used in advanced HF
- Differentiate the mechanisms of action between dobutamine and milrinone
- Summarize components of comprehensive care, assessment, and monitoring
- Prepare a plan for patient education

UNDERSTANDING CARDIAC INFUSION DRUGS

As with all highly specialized infusion therapies, home care nurses who administer cardiac infusion drugs should be experienced in cardiac care and should complete specific agency education and competencies. Inotropic infusion administration in chronic HF management is controversial as it is associated with an increased risk of cardiac death due to arrhythmias. Current HF guidelines recommend the use of long-term inotropic therapy only in those patients with advanced HF refractory to other therapies (Heart Failure Society of America, 2010; Yancy et al., 2013). In a more recent report describing the outcomes of 197 patients discharged on inotropes over a 6-year period, the researchers concluded that survival for those patients who were not candidates for transplant or an LVAD fared better than earlier reports with a median survival of 9 months ($n = 98$ palliative patients; Hashim et al., 2015). For those patients who were awaiting a transplant or LVAD placement, inotropic infusions were evaluated to be effective with 55 of 60 patients successfully maintained on the inotropic infusion until the planned cardiac intervention.

The basic mechanism of inotropic drugs is to increase contractility of the heart in order to increase cardiac output. Dobutamine and milrinone do this through different mechanisms of action (Table 13.1). Positive inotropic drugs are administered as an intermittent or continuous infusion. When administering intermittent infusion regimens, practices vary regarding the frequency and duration of the infusion.

Diuretic therapy is a mainstay in HF management, and loop diuretics (e.g., furosemide and bumetanide) are preferred for most

Table 13.1

Comparison of Dobutamine and Milrinone

	Dobutamine (Dobutrex)	Milrinone (Primacor)
Mechanism of action	A synthetic sympathetic drug. Stimulates beta 1 receptors primarily in cardiac muscle resulting in increased contractility, stroke volume, and cardiac output. Also causes mild beta 2 (vasodilating) and alpha (vasoconstricting) receptor stimulation with little to no effect on peripheral blood vessels	A phosphodiesterase III inhibitor drug. Positive inotrope with vasodilating effect. Causes an increase in intracellular adenosine monophosphate, which stimulates intracellular reactions leading to increased calcium transport. Results in increased ventricular contractility, stroke volume, and cardiac output. Also, relaxation in smooth muscle cells leads to reduced systemic and pulmonary vascular resistance (decreased afterload) through vasodilatation
Dosage and administration	■ Usual dosage 2–20 mcg/kg/min ■ May be given as a continuous or intermittent infusion; lower doses may be safer	■ 0.375–0.750 mcg/kg/min ■ Generally given as an intermittent infusion
Pharmacokinetics	■ Onset of action within 2 minutes; peak drug concentration within 2–10 minutes; half-life about 2 minutes ■ Metabolized in liver; excreted in urine	■ Onset of action within 2–5 minutes; mean half-life 2.4 hours ■ More variable individual response to milrinone ■ Metabolized in liver; excreted in urine
Side effects/ adverse drug effects	■ Increased ventricular arrhythmias, tachycardia, palpitations, angina, headache, and increased blood pressure	■ Thrombocytopenia, arrhythmias, hypotension, angina, and headache

Sources: Gahart, Nazareno, and Ortega (2016); Lyons and Carey (2013).

HF patients (Yancy et al., 2013). To manage fluid volume excess, oral diuretics are temporarily increased. Some patients may become less responsive to diuretic therapy, such as in the context of high dietary sodium intake or in impaired renal function. In such situations, intravenous (IV) diuretic therapy may be administered as needed or on a regular schedule, in conjunction with inotropic therapy (or alone) to maintain fluid volume stability. Subcutaneous administration of furosemide has been reported as successful in diuresis and reduction of hospitalizations in palliative care settings (Farless, Steil, Williams, & Bailey, 2012; Zacharias, Raw, Nunn, Parsons, & Johnson, 2011). The major risk with diuretic administration is electrolyte imbalance. Low potassium and magnesium levels are associated with increased risk of cardiac arrhythmias (Yancy et al., 2013).

Fast Facts in a Nutshell

Home inotropic therapy was found to be safe in pediatric patients who were awaiting a heart transplant. In a retrospective descriptive study, of 106 patients discharged on inotropic infusions (most often milrinone), 85% underwent transplantation. All pediatric patients were fitted with an external automatic defibrillator vest. Adverse outcomes included five line infections (5%), one exit site infection; only two (2%) had clinically significant arrhythmias (Birnbaum et al., 2015).

PATIENT SELECTION CONSIDERATIONS

The complexity, cost, and risks associated with positive inotropic drug infusions demand careful evaluation as patients transition to the home setting. Criteria include:

- The patient and family are motivated, willing, and capable of participating in self-infusion management.
  - Cardiac drug infusions may be continuous or longer intermittent infusions (lasting hours) and are delivered via a central vascular access device (CVAD) using an electronic infusion device. Because the home care nurse does not normally stay in the home for the duration of the infusion, there must be a level of patient or caregiver participation in infusion administration, CVAD-related care, and monitoring.

- A patient in advanced HF should not be left alone during the infusion.
- The caregiver is available to troubleshoot problems in the event of adverse drug reactions, infusion pump problems, or deterioration in condition.
- The patient is clinically stable on the intended home infusion regimen prior to hospital discharge and subsequent home care admission.
  - Any arrhythmias resulting from the infusion are identified and managed.
  - Electrolytes and renal function tests are stable.
  - The patient demonstrates a satisfactory hemodynamic response to the intended therapy (documentation of response required for some insurance payers).
- An appropriate vascular access device (VAD) is selected.
  - A CVAD is required for inotropic infusions; dobutamine is classified as a vesicant drug (Gorski et al., 2017).
  - A peripheral catheter is usually appropriate for patients requiring intermittent diuretic administration. Subcutaneous administration has also been reported.
- Resuscitation status and self-determination are established in the event of an emergency.
  - Potential risks of inotropic infusion therapy should be addressed including the risk of arrhythmias and other adverse outcomes such as central line complications including bloodstream infection (BSI).
  - For patients with advanced HF, families should be counseled that inotropic infusion therapy is palliative, not curative.
- The home environment is safe, clean, with adequate refrigeration space, and the patient has ready access to a telephone.
  - Inotropic drugs and related supplies are generally delivered to the patient home on a weekly basis. Some drugs may require storage in the refrigerator.
- Reimbursement is verified. Private third-party payers vary in coverage.
  - Inotropic infusion therapy may be covered under the durable medical equipment benefit for external infusion pumps under Part B of the Medicare program. Some third-party payers, including Medicare, require very specific documentation as follows:
    - Improvement in hemodynamic parameters such as increase in cardiac index, decrease in pulmonary wedge

pressure, and improvement in level of dyspnea with the inotropic infusion (See Table 13.2 for a description of terminology related to hemodynamics.)

❑ Attempts at discontinuing the inotropic infusion in the hospital

❑ History of repeated hospitalizations for HF exacerbations requiring inotropic support

(Katz et al., 2015; Lyons & Carey, 2013)

Table 13.2

Understanding Hemodynamic Concepts

Cardiac output (CO)	The amount of blood pumped each minute into the aorta by the left ventricle. Normal CO in the adult is approximately 5 L/min. Measured invasively (e.g., pulmonary artery catheter) or noninvasively (e.g., thoracic bioimpedance) CO = Stroke volume × Heart rate
Cardiac index (CI)	CO adjusted for body surface area
Stroke volume	The amount of blood pumped by the left ventricle with each heart beat
Preload	Refers to the resting force of the heart muscle. Determined by the volume in the left ventricle just prior to contraction. Clinical indicators include: Right ventricular preload—reflected by central venous pressure measurement Left ventricular preload—reflected by the pulmonary capillary wedge pressure
Afterload	The resistance to blood flow that is determined by the diameter of the arterioles in the systemic and pulmonary circulation. Vasodilators are used to decrease afterload. Milrinone decreases afterload, making it easier for the heart to pump out blood.
Left ventricular ejection fraction (LVEF)	Reflects the strength of the ventricular contraction. The ratio of the blood ejected from the ventricle in one contraction to the ventricle's total capacity. Normal LVEF is approximately 60%–65%.

COMPREHENSIVE CARE, ASSESSMENT, AND MONITORING

Plan for Home Care and Visit Frequency

- Schedule initial home visits to coincide with the initiation and the discontinuation of an intermittent infusion. Because continuous infusions should not be interrupted as the patient transitions from acute to home care, the home infusion pharmacy typically delivers the infusion medication and infusion pump to the hospital and the home care nurse converts the patient to the home infusion in the hospital just prior to discharge. A home visit is then scheduled shortly after the patient's arrival at his or her home.
- Provide daily (continuous infusion) or twice daily (intermittent infusion) home visits and decrease frequency of home visits as the patient/caregiver learns to perform infusion-related procedures and as patient's cardiac status is stable.
- Continued visit frequency depends upon patient condition, degree of dependence with infusion care, and frequency of physician follow-up.
  - Usual course of home care: Regular home visits to assess cardiac status, monitor response to infusion therapy and overall plan of care
- Consider remote monitoring of vital signs via a telemonitoring system.
  - This is an increasingly common practice for general home care patients with HF (McCaughan, 2017). Telemonitoring should be strongly considered for the patient on inotropic infusions as it allows for at least daily assessment of vital signs, oxygen saturation level, and other data (e.g., patient subjective complaints of level of dyspnea).

Inotropic Drug Administration

- Coordinate the time of the infusion with the referring physician, infusion pharmacy, and the patient.
- Ensure that orders include name(s) of drug, dosage, patient weight (for dosage calculation) route, duration of treatment (e.g., 10 hours per day)/rate of administration.
  - If significant changes in weight occur over time (not attributed to fluid volume excess or deficit), infusion rate should be recalculated. Consult with physician/pharmacist regarding parameters for recalculation (e.g., 5 lb. decrease in weight).

- Verify patient identification and double check infusion rate calculation based on body weight; inotropic drugs are dosed in mcg/kg/min and must be converted to an IV rate in mL/hr; while today, computer programs are most often used to check dosage and infusion rates, it is important for the infusion nurse to be able to check using a manual math formula as follows:

> Multiply patient weight (kg) × drug dose (mcg/kg/min) ×
> 60 min/hr × drug dilution in infusion reservoir/bag (mL/mcg) = IV rate in mL/hr
> (*Note:* convert mg to mcg by multiplying by 1,000)
>
> Example:
>
> 70 kg × 5 mcg/kg/min × 60 min/hr × 250 mL/500,000 mcg
> = 10.5 mL/hr

- Compare order on infusion container/cassette to the physician's order and verify all infusion parameters on syringe (e.g., furosemide) or infusion (e.g., rate, reservoir volume). Because inotropic drugs are high-risk medications, a double-check system should be considered. Although it may not be realistic to send two clinicians to a home with every drug reservoir change, one solution is to have the home care nurse call the pharmacist while in the home and read the infusion pump parameters to confirm the orders and the accuracy of the infusion pump settings.
- Verify patency of VAD.
  - *Never* flush a CVAD with the inotropic medication present in the line because this will result in a bolus of drug; aspirate 2 to 3 mL from the catheter and discard prior to flushing.
  - For continuous infusions, at the time of infusion container/administration set change, consider disconnecting and reconnecting so as to maintain the continuous inotropic infusion without interruption if there are no issues or problems with infusion such as periodic occlusion alarms. Develop an organizational policy for routine assessment of catheter patency (e.g., weekly if no problems).

Assessment and Monitoring

A comprehensive cardiac assessment is completed with each home visit (Fritz & McKenzie, 2015). Monitor the patient for response to the therapy and for potential drug side effects (Table 13.1), paying particular attention to potential signs/symptoms of HF exacerbation:

- Weight: Monitor trend; compare to previous weights on daily log maintained by the patient
- Blood pressure
- Pulse: Apical and radial for both rate and rhythm; assess before starting (intermittent) infusion and 10 to 15 minutes after initiation of infusion
- Breath sounds
- Presence of jugular venous distention
- Edema: Location and grade
- Perfusion: Nailbed color and capillary refill time
- Skin temperature and turgor
- Abdomen for tenderness, changes in abdominal girth
- Mentation and orientation
- Respiratory symptoms such as cough, changes in level of dyspnea/orthopnea
- Urine output and voiding patterns
- Presence of chest pain: When occurred/actions taken
- Presence of any drug side effects or any other subjective complaints by the patient

When a thorough cardiac assessment is performed with each home visit, subtle changes in condition are identified with opportunity for early intervention and reducing the risk for emergent hospitalization. Pay attention to:

- Any signs/symptoms associated with fluid volume excess or signs/symptoms of HF exacerbation such as increased weight or paroxysmal nocturnal dyspnea
  - Establish parameters for reporting changes with the physician.
    - For example, 2 to 3 lb. or more weight gain over 2 to 7 days, increase in heart rate of 10 to 15 beats per minute
  - Oral diuretic therapy may be increased and administered as needed or on a regular schedule, in conjunction with inotropic therapy (or alone) to maintain fluid volume stability.

- Inotropic drug dosage/frequency of infusion therapy may be increased or decreased in the home setting based on patient condition/response.
  - Increase frequency of home visits to assess cardiac status and monitor for response to drug regimen changes.
- Any signs/symptoms of arrhythmias that occur such as increase in irregular beats after starting infusion, complaints of palpitations, chest pain, or evidence of decreasing cardiac output such as decreased BP, urine output, and changes in mentation.
- Laboratory monitoring:
  - Electrolytes and renal function tests are monitored at varying frequency based on patient stability; with frequent increases or changes in diuretic or other drugs, more monitoring is appropriate.
  - B-type natriuretic peptide (BNP) levels:
    - BNP is a cardiac neurohormone released by the ventricles in response to ventricular volume expansion and pressure overload.
    - A BNP level of more than 100 pg/mL is suggestive of HF; patients with advanced HF will have much higher levels.
    - BNP measurement is useful in establishing prognosis and disease severity (Yancy et al., 2013); BNP levels are not routinely monitored.
- Infections were a significant complication and cause of rehospitalizations among patients on inotropic infusions. About 30% of patients suffered an infection, most often bacteremia (Acharya et al., 2016). Attention to aseptic technique during CVAD care and infusion administration is critical.

Psychosocial Considerations

Explore and address potential concerns and issues throughout the course of home care.

- Specific issues may include:
  - Patient/family goals and expected results
  - Quality of life issues
  - Changes in family roles
  - Maintaining activities of daily living
  - Uncertainties of treatment outcomes

- Changes/deterioration in condition and decision making regarding continuation of infusion therapy versus other options such as hospice care
- Financial concerns

PATIENT EDUCATION: KEY POINTS

- Basic HF management: Medications, sodium restriction, fluid restriction (if ordered), and self-monitoring (daily weights)
- Sorting/organizing all infusion supplies and equipment
- Safety precautions related to storage of drug, supplies, and biohazard container
- Concept of aseptic technique and importance in decreasing risk of infection
  - Preparing the infusion container and administration set
  - CVAD-related care
- Setting up and programming the infusion pump/troubleshooting
- Potential complications to report to the physician or nurse
  - Drug side/adverse effects
  - Signs/symptoms of HF exacerbation

TEST YOUR KNOWLEDGE

1. Reimbursement under Medicare requires supporting documentation of improvement in hemodynamic parameters with an inotropic infusion including:
   a. Increased pulmonary wedge pressure
   b. Decreased pulmonary wedge pressure
   c. Decreased cardiac output
   d. Decreased cardiac index
2. The primary pharmacologic action of dobutamine is:
   a. Vasodilatation
   b. Vasoconstriction
   c. Increased contractility
   d. Decreased afterload
3. The half-life of dobutamine is:
   a. 2 to 10 minutes
   b. 2 minutes
   c. 2.4 hours
   d. 5 minutes

4. An adverse reaction associated with milrinone includes:
   a. Hypertension
   b. Tachycardia
   c. Thrombocytopenia
   d. Diarrhea
5. The risk of arrhythmias is associated with which electrolyte imbalance?
   a. High magnesium level
   b. Low magnesium level
   c. High sodium level
   d. Low sodium level
6. Calculate the infusion rate for a dobutamine infusion using the following data: Patient weight 80 kg; dobutamine dosage 5 mcg/kg/min; drug concentration 500,000 mcg in 200 mL.
   a. 10.6 mL/hr
   b. 9.6 mL/hr
   c. 8.6 mL/hr
   d. 11.6 mL/hr

ANSWERS

1. b
2. c
3. b
4. c
5. a
6. b

References

Acharya, D., Sanam, K., Revilla-Martinez, M., Hashim, T., Morgan, C. J., Pamboukian, S. V., . . . Tallaj, J. A. (2016). Infections, arrhythmias, and hospitalizations on home intravenous inotropic therapy. *American Journal of Cardiology, 117*, 952–956.

Birnbaum, B. F., Simpson, K. E., Boschert, T. A., Zheng, J., Wallendorf, M. J., Schectma, K., & Canter, C. E. (2015). Intravenous home inotropic use is safe in pediatric patients awaiting transplantation. *Circulation: Heart Failure, 8*, 64–70.

Ciuksza, M. S., Hebert, R., & Sokos, G. (2015). Fast facts and concepts #283: Use of home inotropes in patients near the end of life. Retrieved from http://www.mypcnow.org/blank-tjctb

Farless, L. B., Steil, N., Williams, B. R., & Bailey, F. A. (2012). Intermittent subcutaneous furosemide: Parenteral diuretic rescue for hospice patients with congestive heart failure resistant to oral diuretic. *American Journal of Hospice & Palliative Medicine, 30*(8), 791–792.

Fritz, D., & McKenzie, P. (2015). Cardiac assessment. *Home Healthcare Now, 33*(9), 466–472.

Gahart, B. L., Nazareno, A. R., & Ortega, M. Q. (2016). *Gahart's 2016 intravenous medications: A handbook for nurses and health professionals* (32nd ed.). St. Louis, MO: Elsevier.

Gorski, L. A., Stranz, M., Cook, L., Joseph, J. M., Kokotis, K., Sabatino-Holmes, P., & VanGosen, L. (2017). Development of an evidence-based list of noncytotoxic vesicant medications and solutions. *Journal of Infusion Nursing, 40*(1), 26–40.

Hashim, T., Sanam, K., Revilla-Martinez, M., Morgan, C. J., Tallaj, J. A., Pamboukian, S. V., . . . Acharya, D. (2015). Clinical characteristics and outcomes of intravenous inotropic therapy in advanced heart failure. *Circulation: Heart Failure, 8*, 880–886.

Heart Failure Society of America. (2010). Section 8: Disease management, advance directives, and end-of-life care in heart failure. *Journal of Cardiac Failure, 16*(6), e98–e114.

Heidenreich, P. A., Albert, N. M., Allen, L. A., Bluemke, D. A., Butler, J., Fonarow G. C., . . . Trogdon, J. G. (2013). Forecasting the impact of heart failure in the United States: A policy statement from the American Heart Association. *Circulation: Heart failure, 6*(3), 606–619.

Katz, J. N., Waters, S. B., Hollis, I. B., & Chang, P. P. (2015). Advanced therapies for end-stage heart failure. *Current Cardiology Reviews, 11*, 63–72.

Lyons, M. G., & Carey, L. (2013). Parenteral inotropic therapy in the home. *Home Healthcare Nurse, 31*(4), 190–204.

McCaughan, A. K. (2017). Home telehealth: Improving care and decreasing costs. In M. D. Harris (Ed.), *Handbook of home healthcare administration* (6th ed., pp. 155–165). Burlington, MA: Jones & Bartlett.

Yancy, C. W., Jessup, M., Bozkurt, B., Butler, J., Casey, D. E., Jr., Drazner, M.H., . . . Wilkoff, B. L. (2013). 2013 ACCF/AHA guideline for the management of heart failure: A report of the American College of Cardiology Foundation/American Heart Association Task Force on Practice Guidelines. *Journal of the American College of Cardiology, 62*, e147–e239.

Zacharias, H., Raw, J., Nunn, A., Parsons, S., & Johnson, M. (2011). Is there a role for subcutaneous furosemide in the community and hospice management of end-stage heart failure? *Palliative Medicine, 25*(6), 658–663.

14

Immunoglobulin Infusion

Immunoglobulin (Ig) therapy is the infusion of concentrated antibodies (i.e, immunoglobulins) into the vascular system. Immunoglobulins may be administered via the intravenous route (IVIg) or subcutaneously (SCIg). They are used in the treatment of both adult and pediatric patients who have an immune system deficiency or impairment and may also be used in the treatment of certain neurological and autoimmune diseases. Primary immunodeficiencies are inherited disorders of immune function that predispose affected persons to an increased rate and severity of infection, immune dysregulation with autoimmune disease and aberrant inflammatory responses, and malignancy. Because the principal clinical manifestation of immune deficiency is increased susceptibility to infection, an overarching goal of Ig replacement therapy is to decrease infections associated with antibody deficiencies. Quality of life is affected and illnesses cause missed days at work, school, and other daily activities of living. The mechanism of action of Ig in treatment of diseases is not well understood but Ig may help to bring a dysregulated immune system back into balance (Immunoglobulin National Society [IgNS], 2015).

Ig preparations are derived from large donor pools of human plasma, as many as 60,000 donors in a batch or lot (IgNS, 2015). Large pools of donors ensure a diversity allowing for recognition of many different antigens. Safety of the Ig product is ensured through careful donor screening for potential risks, inactivation methods to kill pathogens, and clearance methods to remove any pathogens from the product. Although Ig infusions have been relatively free of infectious disease transmission, a reevaluation of preparation processes was required when there was an episode of hepatitis C transmission in the 1990s (IgNS, 2015).

As with all highly specialized infusion therapies, home care nurses who administer Ig products should be experienced and should complete specific agency education and competencies. Furthermore, nurses should be familiar with the IgNS Standards of Practice (2015) that provide detailed guidance for developing organizational policies, procedures, and protocols.

After reading this chapter, the reader will be able to:

- Summarize patient selection criteria
- Differentiate between the benefits/advantages/differences between IV-versus SC-administered Ig
- Describe key aspects of Ig administration
- Summarize components of comprehensive care, assessment, and monitoring
- Prepare a plan for patient education

UNDERSTANDING IMMUNOGLOBULINS: AN OVERVIEW

Immunoglobulins, along with the complement system, are the serum components of the immune system. Other major components include three types of white blood cells—T-lymphocytes, B-lymphocytes, and phagocytes. Each component has a special and essential role in resistance to infection and foreign invasion (Figure 14.1). Produced by B-lymphocytes, immunoglobulins are a family of glycoprotein molecules that are present in the body as solutes in body fluids (plasma and mucous secretions) and are attached to a group of cells in solid tissues; once attached, they inactivate and bind to antigens to facilitate phagocytosis and initiate inflammation by activating the complement cascade (Czaplewski & Vizcarra, 2014). Table 14.1 lists the five classes of immunoglobulins.

IG PRODUCTS

Ig products have different characteristics and these differences are believed to affect the side effect profiles of these products. No head-to-head clinical trials have been done to identify that one product over

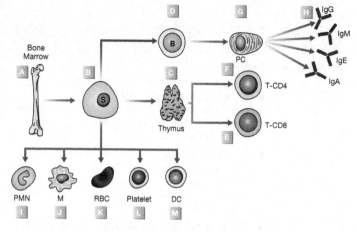

A. Bone marrow: The site in the body where most of the cells of the immune system are produced as immature or stem cells.

B. Stem cells: These cells have the potential to differentiate and mature into the different cells of the immune system.

C. Thymus: An organ located in the chest which instructs immature lymphocytes to become mature T-lymphocytes.

D. B-Cells: These lymphocytes arise in the bone marrow and differentiate into plasma cells which in turn produce immunoglobulins (antibodies).

E. Cytotoxic T-cells: These lymphocytes mature in the thymus and are responsible for killing infected cells.

F. Helper T-cells: These specialized lymphocytes "help" other T-cells and B-cells to perform their functions.

G. Plasma Cells: These cells develop from B-cells and are the cells that make immunoglobulin for the serum and the secretions.

H. Immunoglobulins: These highly specialized protein molecules, also known as antibodies, fit foreign antigens, such as polio, like a lock and key. Their variety is so extensive that they can be produced to match all possible microorganisms in our environment.

I. Neutrophils (Polymorphonuclear PMN Cell): A type of cell found in the blood steam that rapidly ingests microorganisms and kills them.

J. Monocytes: A type of phagocytic cell found in the blood stream which develops into a macrophage when it migrates to tissues.

K. Red Blood Cells: The cells in the blood stream which carry oxygen from the lungs to the tissues.

L. Platelets: Small cells in the blood steam which are important in blood clotting.

M. Dendritic Cells: Important cells in presenting antigen to immune system cells.

Figure 14.1 Cells of the immune system. *Source: Immune System© 2013. Courtesy of the Immune Deficiency Foundation, Towson, MD.*

another is superior. Factors that vary among products include osmolarity, pH, concentration, specific antibody titers, stabilizers (e.g., amino acid based such as glycine or proline vs. sugar based such as fructose, glucose, maltose, sorbitol, or sucrose), sodium content, half-life, and form (lyophilized powder or liquid form; Sun, Teschner, & Yel, 2013). These factors are used in decision making for the most appropriate product for the patient. For example, for the patient with tendency to volume overload, a higher concentration may be used to decrease the overall volume of the infusion. However, increased concentration

Table 14.1

Five Classes of Immunoglobulins	
Immunoglobulins	**Description**
IgG	■ Largest fraction of immunoglobulin ■ Found in the bloodstream and travels to the tissues easily ■ Crosses the placenta, protecting newborn for the first few months after birth
IgA	■ Found in saliva, tears, colostrum, breast milk, intestinal and bronchial secretions ■ Prevents adherence of microorganisms to epithelial surfaces, thus helps resist infections in the respiratory, GI, and urogenital tracts
IgM	■ The first antibodies formed in response to infection ■ Largest molecules ■ Present in the circulation ■ Attacks A and B antigens in the blood leading to transfusion reactions
IgE	■ Trace amounts within blood ■ Responsible for general allergic reactions
IgD	■ Trace amounts within blood ■ Function less understood; antigen recognition

GI, gastrointestinal.

may also increase the risk of reactions (e.g., thrombosis). The use of products with sucrose is avoided in patients with reduced renal function because sucrose is associated with increased risk of renal failure. The amount of IgA content varies as well. This is important because patients with IgA deficiency may develop antibodies to the Ig, which is associated with increased risk for an anaphylactic reaction.

PATIENT SELECTION CONSIDERATIONS

■ Food and Drug Administration (FDA)–approved indications based upon controlled clinical trials include:
   ■ Primary humoral immune deficiency, immune thrombocyto-penic purpura, B-cell chronic lymphocytic leukemia, Kawasaki syndrome, pediatric HIV infection, multifocal motor neuropathy, chronic inflammatory demyelinating

polyneuropathy (IgNS, 2015). Each Ig manufacturer provides specific indications for its product. A list of currently approved Ig products can be found on the Immune Deficiency Foundation at the following website: primaryimmune.org/treatment-information/immunoglobulin-products

- There is evidence for additional use for Ig products with many other immune/antibody-mediated, immunomodulatory, hematological, and dermatologic disorders (e.g., autoimmune hemolytic anemia, graft vs. host disease, dermatomyositis, Guillian–Barré syndrome, myasthenia gravis, and many forms of neuropathy and myopathy; IgNS, 2015; Orange et al., 2006).

- The patient and family are accepting of home infusion therapy.
  - Limitations that preclude home care include mental/physical limitations, substance abuse, psychosocial issues, presence of comorbidities, or need for closer monitoring of the disease process (IgNS, 2015). Other options for Ig infusion include outpatient clinics, physician offices, and ambulatory infusion centers.
  - Insurance may be a factor in choice of settings.

- The patient is clinically stable.
  - The patient is tolerating the Ig without significant reactions and any transient side effects can be managed with premedication(s) (e.g., acetaminophen, diphenhydramine, and hydration, pre-, during, and postinfusion).
  - Review of a detailed history of the patient's comorbid conditions and previous infusion tolerability to Ig can allow for a successful infusion.
  - First doses are generally not administered in the home setting (Younger et al., 2015), although some physicians/organizations may allow for a first dose of SCIg. Always refer to organizational policies and procedures.
    - A change in brand of Ig product or a prolonged interval (more than 8 weeks) between Ig infusions should deem the patient Ig-naïve and at greater risk for adverse events (IgNS, 2015).

- An appropriate vascular access device is planned for Ig administration.
  - Most often, a short peripheral IV catheter is used to administer each IVIg infusion.
  - For patients with poor venous access or compromised vascular integrity, a long-term central venous access device such as an implanted venous access port may be placed if SCIg or other alternatives are not available (IgNS, 2015). Due to the risks of infection and thrombotic complications associated

with central vascular access devices, the American Academy of Allergy, Asthma, and Immunology does not support the use of implantable ports as best practice, unless there are circumstances that require multiple therapies being used to treat the patient (Orange et al., 2006).

- IVIg versus SCIg: Factors that favor SCIg include difficult vascular access, systemic adverse effects with IVIg, or suboptimal health at trough period when IVIg is due, and increased risk for thrombotic events or hemolysis (Bonilla & Duff, 2015).

- The home environment is safe, clean, with adequate refrigeration, adequate light, electricity, and the patient has ready access to a telephone. There is reasonable access to emergency services should a severe reaction occur.

- Reimbursement is verified.
  - Private third-party payers vary in coverage and whether there is access to an additional carve out for specialty pharmacy benefits.
  - The Medicare IVIG Access Act (HR 1845) was signed into law on January 10, 2013, as a 3-year demonstration project to examine the cost-effectiveness of home IVIg infusion administration (Centers for Medicare and Medicaid Services [CMS], 2016; "Medicare Intravenous Immune," *n.d.*). This Medicare law contains a special provision for patients with primary immunodeficiency diseases (PIDD) to receive home infusions of IVIg under Medicare Part B. Medicare will provide a bundled payment under Part B for items and services that are necessary to administer IVIg in the home to enrolled beneficiaries who are not otherwise homebound and are receiving home health care benefits. The demonstration applies *only* to situations where the beneficiary requires IVIg for the treatment of PIDD, or is currently receiving subcutaneous immune globulin to treat PIDD and wishes to switch to intravenous immune globulin. Services are covered through this law through September 30, 2017.

COMPREHENSIVE CARE, ASSESSMENT, AND MONITORING

Plan for Home Care and Visit Frequency

- Unlike most other home infusion therapies and in contrast to SCIg, self-care with IVIg infusions is not the usual goal. Because there is a risk of adverse reactions with each infusion, in most cases the home care nurse administers the IVIg, monitors, and remains in the home for the entire infusion. In one study, treatment outcomes including adherence to therapy and decreased cost of care were improved with nurse-administered home infusion (Luthra, Quimbo, Iyer, & Luo, 2014).

- Schedule home visits to coincide with the time of IVIg administration.
- A typical IVIg home infusion may run over several (e.g., 3–4) hours.
- IVIg infusions are generally administered every 2 to 4 weeks, based on the patient's diagnosis, IgG levels, and response to therapy.
- A follow-up telephone call is recommended 2 to 3 days after infusion to assess for any side effects post-Ig infusion.

Ig Administration

- Ensure that orders include name(s) of Ig product/concentration, dosage (some products recommend a dose adjustment factor), route, frequency of infusion, rate and method of administration.
  - Verify presence of, and orders for use of, a nonexpired anaphylaxis kit (e.g., contents of epinephrine and diphenhydramine) or epinephrine prior to attempting peripheral catheter placement for IVIg or initiating SCIg due to an ongoing risk of reaction (IgNS, 2015).
  - Compare and verify orders of Ig product to physician's order.
- SCIg administration: Advantages of SCIg include a more steady state of IgG levels due to frequency of dosing, less systemic side effects than IVIg, and the ability for total self-care as patients learn how to self-administer infusions.
  - Home care nurses are usually responsible for assisting in the initial training for self-infusion of SCIg infusions (will require several visits based on the patient and the type of product).
  - SCIg infusions are administered at regular intervals from daily up to every 2 weeks (biweekly). Individualize the dose based on the patient's clinical response.
  - The maximum fluid volume of conventional SCIg (10%–20% concentration) per site is usually limited to 15 to 60 mL based on specific product recommendations; this may require infusion into more than one site; up to eight sites may be simultaneously used (IgNS, 2015).

- There is an SC product that uses recombinant human hyaluronidase to facilitate the dispersion and absorption of Ig. The enzyme is administered first then followed by the Ig product within 10 minutes, administered in the upper abdomen or thighs. Always refer to the manufacturer's prescribing information (HyQvia Prescribing Information, 2016).
- In conventional SCIg, the abdomen is preferred by many patients due to adequacy of subcutaneous tissue, but other options include thighs, back of upper arms, and lower back.
- Although there is limited evidence, the practice of aspirating the SC device for absence of a blood return prior to SC infusion is recommended by IgNS (2015) and Infusion Nurses Society (INS; Gorski et al., 2016). There is ongoing discussion of this practice and it has been suggested as a topic for further research.
- Usual administration is via a mechanical or electrical mechanical syringe driver infusion pump but patients may also choose to manually push the SCIg (Shapiro, 2013).
- Local site reactions including swelling, itching, mild to moderate pain, localized warmth, and erythema are common and tend to resolve with 24 to 48 hours after infusion. Note that local reactions tend to diminish over time.
- SC needle length can be a critical factor that may influence tolerability. Children and very thin patients may need a 6-mm needle. Most average-sized patients will use a 9-mm needle. Longer needle lengths (12, 14 mm) may be required for some patients (Younger et al., 2015).

- IVIg administration: Administration methods for IVIg vary based on issues such as infusion rate, concentration (3%–12%), formulations (stabilizers), osmolality, and safety concerns.
  - Ambulatory or stationary electronic infusion devices are preferred for more consistent rate control.
  - Gravity drip may also be used in conjunction with a rate control device such as a manual flow regulator administration set.
  - Many IVIg preparations are in the liquid form, ready for use for room temperature delivery. A few require reconstitution and, following manufacturer's instructions, usually include the use of transfer device.
  - The home care nurse reconstitutes the product just prior to administration (after vascular access is established).
  - Whether reconstituted or liquid form, product may be transferred to a larger IV bag for administration.

- If liquid form is used directly from glass container, vented pump tubing is required.
- Key points related to reconstituting include: use strict aseptic technique; allow adequate time for product to dissolve (varies, less than 5 minutes up to 20 minutes); gently swirl vials to dissolve but *never shake*.
- Some products may recommend use of a filter (most do not).
- Record product lot number and expiration date; this is recommended in the event of a product recall or need to follow up on a product lot.
- Verify patient identification and verify infusion rate on pump.
  - Follow orders/manufacturer's guidelines for rate.
    - Initiate infusion slowly, increasing rate as infusion is tolerated.
    - Too rapid infusion may cause headache and hypotension; symptoms usually resolve with slowing infusion rate.
- Reinforce patient education of when and to whom related signs/symptoms/infusion issues should be reported to the health care professional team (e.g., side effects to physician/pharmacist/nurse vs. infusion pump/ancillary issues to speciality pharmacy).
- General guidelines to prevent and manage adverse reactions (IgNS, 2015):
  - Decrease infusion rate and divide large doses and administer on different days.
  - Consider a product substitution.
  - Change from IVIg to SCIg, if appropriate.
  - In some cases, premedications may be required (e.g., analgesic, antipyretic, and antihistamine prior to IVIg infusion). Steroids may be required for patients with a history of side effects and/or limited product tolerance.
  - Monitor urine output and provide adequate hydration (oral or IV) to reduce risk of inflammatory reactions, thromboembolic events, and renal complications.

Assessment and Monitoring

The patient receiving IVIg therapy is monitored during the infusion for any adverse reactions. Systemic reactions are more common with IVIg and local site reactions more common with SCIg (IgNS, 2015). The most common adverse reactions include headache, nausea, blood pressure changes, flushing, myalgia, arthralgias, urticarial, low-grade fever, chills, chest discomfort, and tachycardia. Significant adverse events include aseptic meningitis, acute renal failure, thrombotic complications, hyperproteinemia, risk of transmitted infection, transfusion-related lung injury (TRALI), hemolytic anemia, and anaphylaxis (IgNS, 2015).

With each infusion, assess/monitor as follows:

- Identify any significant changes in health status prior to each infusion (e.g., respiratory rate, breath sounds, changes in weight, presence of any acute illness, and infection); changes in weight may require a modification of the Ig dose.
- Review laboratory data as appropriate collected prior to the start of the IVIg infusion:
  - Serum IgG trough levels, complete blood count (CBC), serum creatinine, blood urea nitrogen (BUN), electrolytes, and hepatic profile (Czaplewski & Vizcarra, 2014)
- Examine vital signs:
  - Check prior to initiating each IVIg infusion, at regular intervals according to orders/organizational policies, and at the end of the infusion. With long-term stable patients, the frequency for monitoring vital signs may be reduced based on physician discretion.

Fast Facts in a Nutshell

Anaphylaxis is a feared event but is actually quite rare, occurring in less than one in 10,000 infusions (Bonilla & Duff, 2015). The risk is increased in IgA-deficient patients who have developed antibodies against IgA.

- Postinfusion:
  - Flu-like symptoms sometimes occur 2 to 3 days after infusion; premedications may help (e.g., acetaminophen, nonsteroidal anti-inflammatory agent, antimigraine agents, and antihistamine prior to IVIg infusion) to prevent symptoms. These symptoms may be due to antigen–antibody reactions or stabilizers used in the product manufacturing process (Gelfand, 2006).
- Overall response to home therapy:
  - Expected outcome of a decrease in frequency of major and minor infections and decreased hospitalizations
  - Improvement of neurological dysfunction/disability

Fast Facts in a Nutshell

The manufacturing process and attributes of different Ig products are critical for the home care nurse to understand, which may affect tolerability, adverse event profile, and clinical outcomes directly.

Psychosocial Considerations

- Explore and address potential concerns and issues throughout the course of home care.
- Specific issues may include:
  - Lack of understanding of diagnosis and rationale for use of Ig product, which may include the uncertainties related to disease process and outcome of treatment
  - Chronicity of treatment; treatment may be lifelong and issues may include missing work, school or social activities, frequency of infusion, number of needle sticks, lack of awareness of resources, and family /peer support organizations
  - Anxiety due to side effects; anxiety often increases with change in IVIg product, and potential for decreased quality of life
  - Impact on lifestyle; or ability to travel
                                    (IgNS, 2015; Routes et al., 2016)
  - Financial concerns—many companies offer reimbursement assistance programs (e.g., co-pay program); contact manufacturer of product used or Immune Deficiency Foundation (listed in the following)

PATIENT EDUCATION: KEY POINTS

- Brand name and dosage of Ig product prescribed
- Ig actions and side effects
- Potential risks to Ig therapy; may change over time based on comorbidities
- The infusion procedure
- Vascular access device (VAD)–related care (if long-term device)
- Signs and symptoms to report postinfusion.
- Keeping an infusion log to keep track of product used, in maintaining a regular schedule, response to infusions
  - Importance of adherence and regular follow-up with the specialist prescribing the Ig

Fast Facts in a Nutshell

The Immune Deficiency Foundation is an exceptional resource for health care providers, patients, and families. It provides many free patient educational materials for both adults and children and also offer assistance with reimbursement issues, insurance policies, and access to IVIg. Go to primaryimmune.org.

The GBS|CIDP Foundation International is a global nonprofit organization supporting individuals and their families affected by Guillain–Barré syndrome (GBS), chronic inflammatory demyelinating polyneuropathy (CIDP), and related syndromes such as multifocal motor neuropathy (MMN) through a commitment to support, education, research, and advocacy.

Visit www.gbs-cidp.org

TEST YOUR KNOWLEDGE

1. Food and Drug Administration–approved diagnoses for Ig include:
   a. Guillain–Barré
   b. Myasthenia gravis
   c. Immune thrombocyopenic purpura
   d. Multiple sclerosis
2. In a home care study, improved outcomes relative to home IVIg administration include:
   a. Fewer side effects
   b. Better adherence and decreased costs of care
   c. High patient satisfaction
   d. Less psychosocial issues
3. The most common VAD used for IVIg is:
   a. Peripheral IV catheter
   b. Implanted port
   c. Peripherally inserted central catheter
   d. Subcutaneous
4. Immunoglobulins are produced by:
   a. B-lymphocytes
   b. T-lymphocytes
   c. Phagocytes
   d. Neutrophils

5. The risk for anaphylactic reactions is increased in patients with:
   a. IgA deficiency
   b. IgM deficiency
   c. IgE deficiency
   d. IgD deficiency
6. Patients should be advised about the following reaction that can occur a few days after an IVIg infusion:
   a. Blood clots
   b. Flu-like symptoms
   c. Severe headache
   d. Erythema at the IV site

ANSWERS

1. c
2. b
3. a
4. a
5. a
6. b

References

Bonilla, F. A., & Duff, C. A. (2015). Subcutaneous immunoglobulin therapy. *Clinical Focus on Primary Immune Deficiencies, 16,* 1–16.

Centers for Medicare and Medicaid Services. (2016). Medicare intravenous immune globulin (IVIG) demonstration. Retrieved from https://innovation.cms.gov/initiatives/ivig

Czaplewski, L. M., & Vizcarra, C. (2014). Antineoplastic and biologic therapy. In M. Alexander, A. Corrigan, L. A. Gorski, & L. Phillips (Eds.), *Core curriculum for infusion nursing* (5th ed., pp. 258–308). Philadelphia, PA: Lippincott Williams & Wilkins.

Gelfand, E. W. (2006). Differences between IGIV products: Impact on clinical outcome. *International Immunopharmacology, 6*(4), 592–599.

HyQvia Prescribing Information. (2016). Retrieved from http://www.shirecontent.com/PI/PDFs/HYQVIA_USA_ENG.pdf

Immune Deficiency Foundation. (2013). *Patient and family handbook for primary immunodeficiency diseases* (5th ed.). Towson, MD: Author.

Immunoglobulin National Society. (2015). *IgNS nursing standards of practice.* Woodland Hills, CA: Author.

Luthra, R., Quimbo, R., Iyer, R., & Luo, M. (2014). An analysis of intravenous immunoglobulin site of care: Home versus hospital. *American Journal of Pharmacy Benefits, 6,* e41–e49.

Medicare Intravenous Immune Globulin Demonstration. (n.d.). [Fact sheet]. Retrieved from https://innovation.cms.gov/Files/fact-sheet/IVIG_Fact-Sheet.pdf

Orange, J. S., Hossny, E. M., Weiler, C. R., Ballow, M., Berger, M., Bonilla, F. A., . . . Cunningham-Rundles, C. (2006). Use of intravenous immunoglobulin in human disease: A review of evidence by members of the Primary Immunodeficiency Committee of the American Academy of Allergy, Asthma and Immunology. *Journal of Allergy and Clinical Immunology, 117*(4, Suppl.), S525–S553.

Routes, J., Costa-Carvalho, B. T., Grimbacher, B., Paris, K., Ochs, H. D., Filipovich, A., . . . Li-McLeod, J. (2016). Health-related quality of life and health resource utilization in patients with primary immunodeficiency disease prior to and following 12 months of immunoglobulin G treatment. *Journal of Clinical Immunology, 36*, 450–461.

Shapiro, R. S. (2013). Subcutaneous immunoglobulin: Rapid push vs. infusion pump in pediatrics. *Pediatric Allergy and Immunology, 24*(1), 49–53.

Sun, A., Teschner, W., & Yel, L. (2013). Improving patient tolerance in immunoglobulin treatment: Focus on stabilizer effects. *Expert Reviews in Clinical Immunology, 9*(6), 577–587.

Younger, M. E., Blouin, W., Duff, C., Epland, K. B., Murphy, E., & Sedlak, D. (2015). Subcutaneous immunoglobulin replacement therapy: Ensuring success. *Journal of Infusion Nursing, 38*(1), 7–79.

15

Other Home Infusion Therapies

The purpose of this chapter is to provide an overview of some less common, but often home-administered infusion therapies that do not fall under the broad headings of the previous chapters. These infusion drug therapies are associated with uncommon or rare diseases and the infusion drugs may be associated with significant adverse effects. In almost every case, these drugs are not administered as first doses in the home setting. Patients who do not experience significant adverse reactions or side effects may be transitioned to home infusion. Some of the drugs require reconstitution in the home and it is important to read the specific drug product inserts prior to preparing the infusion. The home care nurse should have an excellent understanding of the disease processes and the specific infusion therapies prior to managing these unusual patient populations. Additional resources, as available, are included in each section. It is important to note that this chapter is not inclusive of all possible home-administered therapies. As the practice of home infusion therapy grows, as the safety profile for home-administered medications is established, and as new medications are approved by the Food and Drug Administration (FDA), this list will grow. It is not uncommon for home care organizations to receive referrals for infusion medications that are not usual. Before accepting a referral for an infusion therapy, it is important to investigate the safety of the infusate, the risks especially as they relate to a home infusion, and the rationale for home administration. This requires interprofessional collaboration between the physician, the pharmacist, and the nursing organization. Patient safety is paramount in such decision making.

After reading this chapter, the reader will be able to:

- Identify indications for other infusion drugs that may be home administered
- Discuss key aspects of assessment and monitoring of these infusion drugs

ALPHA₁-PROTEINASE INHIBITOR (ARALAST NP, PROLASTIN-C, GLASSIA, ZEMAIRA)

Description

- Purified human alpha₁-proteinase inhibitor, which is also known as alpha₁-antitrypsin (AAT). Product is prepared from large pools of human plasma; manufacturing processes are used to reduce risk of potential viral transmission.

Indications

- Long-term chronic replacement therapy for the treatment of AAT deficiency, a hereditary condition that results in chronic obstructive pulmonary disease.
- AAT protects lungs from a natural enzyme (neutrophil elastase) that fights bacteria and cleans up dead lung tissue; this enzyme can also damage the lungs if not neutralized by AAT.
- Symptoms are primarily shortness of breath with activity, decreased exercise tolerance, and wheezing beginning between 20 and 40 years of age.
- AAT deficiency is diagnosed with a blood test.
- The goal of treatment is to slow or stop the progression of lung destruction by replacing the deficient protein. The therapy cannot restore lost lung function and it is not considered a cure. There is some evidence that augmentation therapy can reduce the frequency and severity of pulmonary exacerbations. (Alpha 1 Foundation: www.alpha1.org).

Infusion Guidelines

- Prolastin-C: Manufacturer recommends immunization against hepatitis B prior to initiating treatment.

- It is administered as an IV infusion over 30 to 60 minutes, most often as a gravity infusion.
- It is usually administered with a peripheral venous catheter; started with each dose.
  - Establish venous access prior to reconstitution (due to high drug cost, cannot risk inability to infuse due to IV placement issues).
- Alpha$_1$-proteinase inhibitor is a lyophilized powder or ready-to-use solution.
  - The powder is reconstituted in the patient's home just prior to administration; several vials may be used for one dose; reconstituted alpha$_1$-proteinase inhibitor is pooled into an empty IV container for infusion. Follow package insert instructions.
  - Key points related to reconstituting: Use strict aseptic technique, allow adequate time for product to dissolve, may gently roll vial but *never shake*.

(Gahart, Nazareno, & Ortega, 2016)

Monitoring/Adverse Reactions

- It is generally well tolerated.
- Adverse symptoms are infrequent but may include pharyngitis, headache, cough, delayed fever, lightheadedness, and dizziness.
- Alpha$_1$-proteinase inhibitor is contraindicated in persons with IgA deficiencies who have developed antibodies against IgA; anaphylactic reactions could occur.

PATIENT EDUCATION: KEY POINTS

- Indications and rationale for treatment
- Signs/symptoms of adverse reactions to report
- Lifelong treatment
- Importance of therapy adherence and keeping physician (MD)/laboratory appointments for regular follow-up
- Patient (and clinician) resource: Alpha 1 Foundation: www.alpha1.org

DEFEROXAMINE MESYLATE (DESFERAL)

Description

- An iron chelating agent; binds with iron to form ferrioxamine, a chelate that prevents iron from entering into further chemical reactions
- Removes iron from free serum iron, ferritin, and transferrin
- Also used in the chelation of aluminum in patients with chronic renal failure

Indications

- In the home care setting, deferoxamine is used for the treatment of chronic iron overload often associated with patients who have a history of repeated blood transfusions (e.g., with sickle cell anemia, aplastic anemia, chronic hemolytic anemia) or secondary hemochromotosis, an iron overload disorder.
- Without treatment, excessive iron accumulation results in joint problems, decreased liver function, cardiac damage, and endocrine disorders.

Infusion Guidelines

- Routes include subcutaneous and intravenous infusions
- Most often given as a subcutaneous infusion of 1 to 2 g per day (adult dose) over 8 to 24 hours; dosage rate should not exceed 15 mg/kg/hr; weight-based dosage adjustments in children (dosage should not exceed 40 mg/kg/d)
- Requires an infusion pump
- Intermittent infusions often administered during nighttime hours for patient convenience (Eckes, 2011)
- Resource: www.drugs.com/pro/deferoxamine.html#fcf7eafe -cf86-4e12-b6a8-83cd2f0d103b

Monitoring/Adverse Reactions

- Hearing and visual problems can occur.
- Hearing and vision are regularly tested during chronic therapy.
- Side effects associated with too rapid infusion include abdominal discomfort, allergic type reactions, diarrhea, fever, hypotension, and leg cramps.

- Laboratory monitoring:
    - Serum iron concentration
    - Serum ferritin levels

PATIENT EDUCATION: KEY POINTS

- Indications and rationale for treatment
- Signs/symptoms of adverse reactions to report
- Turns urine color reddish color
- Importance of therapy adherence and keeping MD/laboratory appointments for regular follow-up (Eckes, 2011)
- Infusion-related teaching: Subcutaneous site access, infusion pump and related management—patients usually become completely independent with infusions

FACTOR REPLACEMENT FOR HEMOPHLIA: RECOMBINANT PRODUCTS

Description

- Most often factor replacement products used are derived from recombinant DNA rather than processed from donated plasma. This allows for home administration. Most patients will learn to self-administer.

Indications

- Hemophilia A is a deficiency of coagulation factor VIII that occurs in about 1:10,000 males (Hitch, 2013). Factor VIII replacement either is used routinely for patients with severe hemophilia or may be used situationally in moderate to mild cases, such as patients undergoing prophylactic therapy with planned surgery or with a traumatic event.
- Hemophilia B is a deficiency of coagulation factor IX that occurs in about 1:50,000 males (Hitch, 2013).

Infusion Guidelines

- Factor replacement doses are in units and each lot contains a different number of units per vial. The cost of factor replacement is high and dosages are usually prescribed as a range as it is unlikely to find a vial with an exact number of units to match the prescribed weight-based dosage (Hitch, 2013).

- It is administered by slow IV push infusion, no faster than 10 mL/min (Gahart et al., 2016). Always refer to specific manufacturer's directions.
- Dosing varies based on treatment versus prophylaxis, type of bleeding episodes (minor, moderate, or major), or type of surgery (minor or major).
- It is packaged in kits that include a vial of factor (powder), a diluent, and a mixing device; most come with a built-in filter. Sometimes, a steel needle IV device is included in the kit.
- It is generally supplied by the blood center and stored in refrigerator or at room temperature (as directed by the manufacturer); shelf-life up to 2 years.

Monitoring/Adverse Reactions

- Most common side effects include headache, dizziness, nausea, rash, pain in extremity, and oral paresthesia depending upon the specific product.
- Factor VIII: The most frequently reported adverse reactions in clinical trials were headache, pyrexia, and pruritus (www.kovaltry-us.com/hcp).
- Factor IX: Most common side effects include headache, dizziness, rash, hives, injection site reactions/pain, and nausea (www.drugs.com/monograph/factor-ix-recombinant.html).
- Patients can develop antibodies to replacement factor, making it more difficult to control bleeding. This may require higher doses or a bypassing agent that allows clotting to occur without factor VIII or IX (Hitch, 2013).

PATIENT EDUCATION: KEY POINTS

- Goal: self-administration
- How to administer including how to access peripheral vein for infusion
- Side effects to report (difficulty breathing, hives, itching, chest tightness, and wheezing) and to discontinue use
- Lack of clinical response (bleeding)

IMIGLUCERASE (CEREZYME), TALIGLUCERASE ALFA (ELELYSO), VELAGLUCERASE ALFA (VPRIV)

Description

- Facilitates the release of lipid glucocerebrosides in tissues for patients with Gaucher disease.

Indications

- Long-term replacement therapy for the treatment of Gaucher disease, a hereditary metabolic storage disorder that results in a deficiency of the lysosomal enzyme glucocerebrosidase
  - When this enzyme is not present, there is an accumulation of lipid glucocerebrosides in tissues.
  - Gaucher disease affects all ethnic and racial backgrounds but is most prevalent in the eastern European Jewish population.
  - The disease presents with hepatosplenamegaly, anemia, thrombocytopenia, pathologic fractures, and bone pain.

Infusion Guidelines

- Administered as an IV infusion over 1 to 2 hours, most often as a gravity infusion
- Refer to specific manufacturer guidelines for dosing and preparation:
  - VPRIV®: www.elelyso.com
  - Cerezyme®: www.cerezyme.com/patients/treatment_with_cerezyme.aspx
  - ELEYSO®: www.vpriv.com
- Infusion frequency ranges from three times per week to once per month
- Usually administered with a peripheral venous catheter; started with each dose
  - Establish venous access prior to reconstitution (due to high drug cost, cannot risk inability to infuse due to IV placement issues).
  - Key points related to reconstituting: Use strict aseptic technique, allow adequate time for product to dissolve, may gently roll vial but *never shake*.
- Administration set flushed with normal saline at completion of infusion to insure that all of drug is administered

Monitoring/Adverse Reactions

- Adverse reactions are infrequent.
- If signs/symptoms of nausea, vomiting, chills, itching, or rash occur, stop infusion and notify MD; these may be signs of an allergic reaction and could progress to become more severe. Antibodies to Cerezyme can develop, especially during first year of treatment. Patients are generally monitored for IgG antibodies during that time. Premedications such as antihistamines and corticosteroids, as well as a decrease in IV rate, may be used.

PATIENT EDUCATION: KEY POINTS

- Indications and rationale for treatment
- Signs/symptoms of adverse reactions to report
- Lifelong treatment
- Importance of therapy adherence and keeping MD/laboratory appointments for regular follow-up
  - No longer than 1 month between treatments
- Resource: National Gaucher Foundation: www.gaucherdisease.org

INFLIXIMAB (REMICADE)

Description

- It is a monoclonal antibody that acts in the same way as natural antibodies by binding and inactivating an antigen—in this case, tumor necrosis factor-α (TNF-α). TNF-α is recognized as a key factor in the development of a number of immune-mediated diseases such as rheumatoid arthritis and Crohn's disease.

Indications

- Crohn's disease, pediatric Crohn's disease, ulcerative colitis, pediatric ulcerative colitis, rheumatoid arthritis in conjunction with methotrexate, ankylosing spondylitis, psoriatic arthritis, and plaque psoriasis

Infusion Guidelines

- Administered as an IV infusion over not less than 2 hours; usually titrated at slowly increasing rates via a programmable infusion pump to reduce the risk for infusion reactions

- Filter using a 1.2-μm filter or less
- Usually administered with a peripheral venous catheter; started with each dose
  - Establish venous access prior to reconstitution (due to high drug cost, cannot risk inability to infuse due to IV placement issues).
- Infliximab is supplied as a lyophilized powder in 100 mg vials; preparation instructions are in package insert.
  - The powder is reconstituted with sterile water in the patient's home just prior to administration; several vials may be used for one dose.
  - Total reconstituted dose is diluted in a bag of 250 mL of 0.9% normal saline; the volume of the reconstituted drug is withdrawn from the 250 mL bag prior to adding drug to IV bag.
  - Key points related to reconstituting: Use strict aseptic technique, allow adequate time for product to dissolve (5 minutes), may gently roll vial but *never shake*.

Monitoring/Adverse Reactions

- Adverse reactions are usually mild to moderate, decrease over the course of therapy, and do not affect the patient's clinical response.
- Monitor vital signs before, during, and up to 30 minutes postinfusion.
- If signs/symptoms of fever, chills, pruritus, or unusual feelings are experienced by the patient, stop infusion and notify MD. Antibodies to infliximab can develop. Premedications are used for patients with a history of infusion-related reactions including diphenhydramine, acetaminophen, and prednisone.
- Other adverse reactions: May increase risk of severe infections, may cause worsening of heart failure, and is contraindicated with this patient population.
- Most common side effects are respiratory infections, headache, coughing, and stomach pain.
- Postinfusion reactions up to 2 hours after infusion are fever, chills, chest pain, low/high blood pressure, shortness of breath, rash, and itching.
- Drug references:
  - www.remicade.com
  - www.remicade.com/shared/product/remicade/medication-guide.pdf

PATIENT EDUCATION: KEY POINTS

- Infliximab—indications and rationale for treatment
- Signs/symptoms of adverse reactions to report
- Chronic treatment
- Importance of therapy adherence and keeping MD/laboratory appointments for regular follow-up
- Resource: Remicade Medication Guide: www.remicade.com/shared/product/remicade/medication-guide.pdf

METHYLPREDNISOLONE (SOLU-MEDROL)

Description

- An adrenocorticosteroid with metabolic and anti-inflammatory effects
- Greater anti-inflammatory effect than prednisolone with less sodium and water retention and less potassium and calcium excretion
- Used primarily for anti-inflammatory and immunosuppresive effects

Indications

- Intermittent infusions of methylprednisone may be administered at home to patients with exacerbations of multiple sclerosis.

Infusion Guidelines

- May be administered as short intravenous infusion (less than 30 minutes) or less often, IV push over several minutes
- Usually administered with a peripheral venous catheter; started with each dose
- Dosage varies widely

Monitoring/Adverse Reactions

- It may increase blood pressure.
- Side effects associated with too rapid infusion include abdominal discomfort, allergic type reactions, diarrhea, fever, hypotension, and leg cramps.
- Laboratory monitoring:

- Serum electrolytes
- Serum glucose, especially in patients with diabetes

PATIENT EDUCATION: KEY POINTS

- Indications and rationale for treatment
- Signs/symptoms of adverse reactions to report such as edema, weight gain, gastric signs/symptoms, tarry stools, weakness, nausea, and vomiting (Gahart et al., 2016)
- May mask signs/symptoms of infection
- Importance of therapy compliance and keeping MD/laboratory appointments for regular follow-up

PULMONARY HYPERTENSION INFUSION THERAPIES:TREPROSTINAL, EPOPROSTENOL (FLOLAN), ROOM TEMPERATURE STABLE EPOPROSTENOL (VELETRI®)

Description

- These are potent vasodilators with effects on the systemic and pulmonary arteries; decreases right and left ventricular afterload.
- Each of these drugs is available and provided directly only from specialty pharmacies (Accredo Health Group, Inc., and CVS Caremark) that provide a team of clinical pharmacists and nurses (www.phassociation.org).

Indications

- Long-term treatment of primary pulmonary hypertension (PPH), a life-threatening illness
- Symptoms: shortness of breath, dizziness, fatigue, angina, palpitations, syncope, edema, dry cough, and Raynaud's phenomenon

Infusion Guidelines

- Treprostinil: Administered as an SC or IV infusion via a programmable infusion pump. It is stable at room temperature for at least 48 hours. The half-life of treprostinil is about 4.5 hours. Stopping treprostinil can be fatal when done abruptly.

- Epoprostenol (Flolan): Epoprostenol is not stable at room temperature. It requires refrigeration for storage and needs to be kept cold with ice while being infused; small cold packs are used in the pouch that houses the infusion reservoir and the pump.
- Room temperature stable epoprostenol (Veletri):
  - Require an ambulatory electronic infusion pump; back-up infusion pump is kept in home.
  - Reconstituted in the home; use only diluent provided by manufacturer (glycine buffer).
  - Fact sheets for each type of treatment are available from the Pulmonary Hypertension Association (www.phassociation .org/Treatments).

Monitoring/Adverse Reactions

- Infusion cannot be interrupted for longer than 2 to 3 minutes as abrupt discontinuation can cause a rapid return of symptoms; access to a back-up infusion pump is necessary (Gahart et al., 2016).
- Most common side effects include flushing, dizziness, itching, muscle/joint pain, headache, jaw pain, nausea, vomiting, diarrhea, low blood pressure—these symptoms are dose limiting.

PATIENT EDUCATION: KEY POINTS

- Indications and rationale for treatment
- Self-administration; patients will not be discharged home unless independent with managing infusions
- Signs/symptoms of adverse reactions to report
- Aseptic technique, drug reconstitution, infusion pump management, ordering and maintaining supplies
- The availability of a "mixing partner"—a person who can perform all infusion-related tasks in the event the patient is not able to do this
- Lifelong therapy
- Importance of therapy adherence and keeping MD/laboratory appointments for regular follow-up
- Resource: Pulmonary Hypertension Association: www.phasso ciation.org

TEST YOUR KNOWLEDGE

1. Adverse reactions associated with deferoxamine include:
   a. Nephrotoxicity
   b. Severe diarrhea
   c. Low blood pressure
   d. Hearing/visual problems
2. Imiglucerase:
   a. Replaces alpha$_1$-proteinase inhibitors
   b. Binds and inactivates tumor necrosis factor
   c. Facilitates the release of lipid glucocerebrosides
   d. Provides anti-inflammatory effects
3. Premedications such as diphenhydramine or acetaminophen may be required when administering this infusion therapy:
   a. Imiglucerase
   b. Factor replacement
   c. Deferoxamine
   d. Methylprednisolone
4. This infusion drug must be kept cold during the infusion; small cold packs are used in the pouch that houses the infusion reservoir and the pump:
   a. Alpha$_1$-proteinase inhibitor
   b. Imiglucerase
   c. Epoprostenol
   d. Treprostinil

ANSWERS

1. d
2. c
3. a
4. c

References

Eckes, E. J. (2011). Chelation therapy for iron overload. *Journal of Infusion Nursing, 34*(6), 374–380.

Gahart, B. L., Nazareno, A. R., & Ortega, M. Q. (2016). *Gahart's 2016 intravenous medications: A handbook for nurses and health professionals* (32nd ed.). St. Louis, MO: Elsevier.

Hitch, D. (2013). What every nurse should know about hemophilia. *American Nurse Today, 8*(3), 22–26.

Index

Page numbers followed by "*f*" indicate a figure; those followed by "*t*" indicate a table.

Printed in the United States
By Bookmasters